Left Ventricular Summit

Editors

PASQUALE SANTANGELI
FERMIN C. GARCIA
LUIS C. SÁENZ

CARDIAC ELECTROPHYSIOLOGY CLINICS

www.cardiacEP.theclinics.com

Consulting Editors
JORDAN M. PRUTKIN
EMILY P. ZEITLER

March 2023 • Volume 15 • Number 1

ELSEVIER

1600 John F. Kennedy Boulevard • Suite 1800 • Philadelphia, Pennsylvania, 19103-2899

http://www.theclinics.com

CARDIAC ELECTROPHYSIOLOGY CLINICS Volume 15, Number 1
March 2023 ISSN 1877-9182, ISBN-13: 978-0-323-98725-7

Editor: Joanna Gascoine
Developmental Editor: Hannah Almira Lopez

Cardiac Electrophysiology Clinics (ISSN 1877-9182) is published quarterly by Elsevier Inc., 360 Park Avenue South, New York, NY 10010-1710. Months of issue are March, June, September, and December. Subscription prices are $259.00 per year for US individuals, $464.00 per year for US institutions, $272.00 per year for Canadian individuals, $524.00 per year for Canadian institutions, $331.00 per year for international individuals, $562.00 per year for international institutions and $100.00 per year for US, Canadian and international students/residents. To receive student/resident rate, orders must be accompanied by name of affiliated institution, date of term, and the signature of program/residency coordinator on institution letterhead. Orders will be billed at individual rate until proof of status is received. Foreign air speed delivery is included in all Clinics subscription prices. All prices are subject to change without notice. **POST-MASTER:** Send address changes to Cardiac Electrophysiology Clinics, Elsevier Health Sciences Division, Subscription Customer Service, 3251 Riverport Lane, Maryland Heights, MO 63043. **Customer Service: 1-800-654-2452 (US and Canada). From outside of the US and Canada, call 314-477-8871. Fax: 314-447-8029. E-mail: JournalsCustomer-Service-usa@elsevier.com (for print support); JournalsOnlineSupport-usa@elsevier.com (for online support).**

Reprints. For copies of 100 or more of articles in this publication, please contact the Commercial Reprints Department, Elsevier Inc., 360 Park Avenue South, New York, NY 10010-1710. Tel.: 212-633-3874; Fax: 212-633-3820; E-mail: reprints@elsevier.com.

Cardiac Electrophysiology Clinics is covered in *MEDLINE/PubMed (Index Medicus)*.

Contributors

CONSULTING EDITORS

JORDAN M. PRUTKIN, MD, MHS
Professor of Medicine, Division of Cardiology, University of Washington, Seattle, Washington, USA

EMILY P. ZEITLER, MD, MHS
Dartmouth Health, The Dartmouth Institute, Lebanon, New Hampshire, USA; Assistant Professor of Medicine, Dartmouth Geisel School of Medicine, Hanover, New Hampshire, USA

EDITORS

PASQUALE SANTANGELI, MD, PhD
Associate Section Head, Cardiac Electrophysiology Director of the VT Program Cleveland Clinic, Cleveland, Ohio, USA

FERMIN C. GARCIA, MD
Section of Cardiac Electrophysiology, Hospital of the University of Pennsylvania, Philadelphia, Pennsylvania, USA

LUIS C. SÁENZ, MD
Cardiologist and Electrophysiologist, Director Internacional Arrhythmia Center, Fundación Cardio Infantil-Instituto de Cardiología, Bogotá, Colombia

AUTHORS

ISABELLA ALVIZ, MD
Montefiore Medical Center, Albert Einstein College of Medicine, Bronx, New York, USA

FRANK BOGUN, MD
Electrophysiology Section, Division of Cardiovascular Medicine, Department of Internal Medicine, University of Michigan, Ann Arbor, Michigan, USA

JASON S. BRADFIELD, MD
UCLA Cardiac Arrhythmia Center, UCLA Cardiovascular Interventional Programs, Department of Medicine, David Geffen School of Medicine at UCLA, UCLA Health System, Los Angeles, California, USA

SHIH-ANN CHEN, MD
Heart Rhythm Center and Division of Cardiology, Department of Medicine, Taipei Veterans General Hospital, Taipei, Taiwan; Cardiovascular Center, Taichung Veterans General Hospital, Taichung, Taiwan

FA-PO CHUNG, MD, Phd
Heart Rhythm Center and Division of Cardiology, Department of Medicine, Taipei Veterans General Hospital, Department of Medicine, National Yang Ming Chiao Tung University, School of Medicine, Taipei, Taiwan

LUIGI DI BIASE, MD, PhD, FHRS
Section Head Electrophysiology, Director of Arrhythmia Services, Professor of Medicine, Montefiore Medical Center, Albert Einstein College of Medicine, Bronx, New York, USA

JUAN CARLOS DIAZ, MD
Arrhythmia and electrhophysiology service, Clinica Las Vegas, Grupo Quiron Salud;

Universidad CES School of Medicine, Medellin, Colombia, USA

ANDRES ENRIQUEZ, MD
Division of Cardiology, Queen's University, Kingston, Ontario, Canada

THOMAS FLAUTT, DO
Division of Cardiac Electrophysiology, Department of Cardiology, Houston Methodist DeBakey Heart and Vascular Center, Houston Methodist Hospital, Houston, Texas, USA

KOJI FUKUZAWA, MD, PhD
Section of Arrhythmia, Division of Cardiovascular Medicine, Department of Internal Medicine, Kobe University Graduate School of Medicine

PIOTR FUTYMA, MD, PhD
Medical College, University of Rzeszów, St. Joseph's Heart Rhythm Center, Rzeszów, Poland

MOHAMED GABR, MD
Montefiore Medical Center, Albert Einstein College of Medicine, Bronx, New York, USA

MARIA GAMERO, MD
Montefiore Medical Center, Albert Einstein College of Medicine, Bronx, New York, USA

MICHAEL GRUSHKO, MD
Montefiore Medical Center, Albert Einstein College of Medicine, Bronx, New York, USA

GUSTAVO S. GUANDALINI, MD
Assistant Professor of Clinical Medicine, Section of Cardiac Electrophysiology, Hospital of the University of Pennsylvania–Pavilion, Philadelphia, Pennsylvania, USA

MATTHEW G. HANSON, MD
Division of Cardiology, Queen's University, Kingston, Ontario, Canada

JUSTIN HAYASE, MD
UCLA Cardiac Arrhythmia Center, UCLA Cardiovascular Interventional Programs, Department of Medicine, David Geffen School of Medicine at UCLA, UCLA Health System, Los Angeles, California, USA

SURAJ KRISHNAN, MD
Montefiore Medical Center, Albert Einstein College of Medicine, Bronx, New York, USA

JACKSON J. LIANG, DO
Electrophysiology Section, Division of Cardiovascular Medicine, Department of Internal Medicine, University of Michigan, Ann Arbor, Michigan, USA

AUNG LIN, MD
Montefiore Medical Center, Albert Einstein College of Medicine, Bronx, New York, USA

YENN-JIANG LIN, MD, PhD
Heart Rhythm Center and Division of Cardiology, Department of Medicine, Taipei Veterans General Hospital, Department of Medicine, National Yang Ming Chiao Tung University, School of Medicine, Taipei, Taiwan

MARTA LORENTE, MD
Montefiore Medical Center, Albert Einstein College of Medicine, Bronx, New York, USA

SHUMPEI MORI, MD, PhD
UCLA Cardiac Arrhythmia Center, UCLA Cardiovascular Interventional Programs, Department of Medicine, David Geffen School of Medicine at UCLA, UCLA Health System, Los Angeles, California, USA

ANDREA NATALE, MD, FHRS
Texas Cardiac Arrhythmia Institute, St. David's Medical Center, Austin, Texas, USA

ALEJANDRO JIMENEZ RESTREPO, MD, FRACP, FHRS
Cardiac Electrophysiologist, Marshfield Clinic Health System, Marshfield, Wisconsin, USA; Adjunct Associate Professor of Medicine, University of Maryland School of Medicine

JORGE ROMERO, MD, FHRS
Montefiore Medical Center, Albert Einstein College of Medicine, Bronx, New York, USA

LUIS CARLOS SAENZ MORALES, MD, FHRS
Director, International Arrhythmia Center, Fundacion CardioInfantil, Instituto de Cardiologia, Bogota, Colombia

WILLIAM H. SAUER, MD
Cardiac Arrhythmia Service, Brigham and Women's Hospital, Boston, Massachusetts, USA

YASUHIRO SHIRAI, MD, PhD
Department of Cardiology, Disaster Medical
Center, Tokyo, Japan

KALYANAM SHIVKUMAR, MD, PhD
UCLA Cardiac Arrhythmia Center, UCLA
Cardiovascular Interventional Programs,
Department of Medicine, David Geffen School
of Medicine at UCLA, UCLA Health System,
Los Angeles, California, USA

AADHAVI SRIDHARAN, MD, PhD
UCLA Cardiac Arrhythmia Center, UCLA
Cardiovascular Interventional Programs,
Department of Medicine, David Geffen
School of Medicine at UCLA, UCLA Health
System, Los Angeles, California,
USA

ABIGAIL LOUISE D. TE-ROSANO, MD
Heart Rhythm Center and Division of
Cardiology, Department of Medicine, Taipei
Veterans General Hospital, Taipei, Taiwan; HB
Calleja Heart and Vascular Institute, St. Luke's
Medical Center, Quezon City, Philippines

CRISTIAN CAMILO TOQUICA, MD
Montefiore Medical Center, Albert Einstein
College of Medicine, Bronx, New York,
USA

MIGUEL VALDERRÁBANO, MD, PhD
Director, Division of Cardiac Electrophysiology,
Department of Cardiology, Houston Methodist
DeBakey Heart and Vascular Center, Houston
Methodist Hospital, Houston, Texas, USA

ALEJANDRO VELASCO, MD
Montefiore Medical Center, Albert Einstein
College of Medicine, Bronx, New York, USA

TAKUMI YAMADA, MD, PhD
Professor of Medicine, Cardiovascular
Division, University of Minnesota, Minneapolis,
Minnesota, USA

FENGWEI ZOU, MD
Montefiore Medical Center, Albert Einstein
College of Medicine, Bronx, New York, USA

Contents

15% of idiopathic outflow tract ventricular arrhythmias. Direct epicardial ablation of outflow tract ventricular arrhythmias arising from the LVS is successful only in a minority of patients because of close proximity to the coronary artery or thick epicardial fat. Therefore, alternative strategies should be prioritized before performing epicardial approach. When performed, electrocardiogram characteristics suggestive of the site of origin to be the accessible area within the LVS needs be evaluated to avoid ineffective epicardial approach.

Idiopathic ventricular arrhythmias (VA), particularly left ventricular outflow tract (LVOT) VA accounts for up to 10% of all VAs referred for ablative therapy. In addition to being infrequent, its intricate anatomy and its pathophysiology make catheter ablation (CA) of these arrhythmias a challenge even for experts. In this scenario, detailed right ventricular outflow tract as well as LVOT electroanatomic mapping including epicardial mapping are essential. In this article, we will emphasize our approach toward the CA technique used for LVOT VA, particularly IVS and/or LVS VA originating from intramural foci, along with its acute and long-term efficacy and safety.

Left ventricular outflow tract arrhythmias that fail endocardial mapping and ablation have traditionally been labeled as originating from the epicardial left ventricular summit. Although these sometimes can be targeted from the epicardial surface of the left ventricular ostium, such approach poses significant technical challenges. A significant proportion of such arrhythmias, however, exhibit intramyocardial origin, demonstrated by mapping intraseptal branches of the anterior interventricular vein, and henceforth defined as the basal superior intraseptal space.

Most idiopathic ventricular arrhythmias (VAs) originate from the outflow tract (OT) region and can be targeted with ablation either from the endocardial aspect of the right and left ventricular outflow tracts or from the aortic sinuses of Valsalva. It is important to exclude scar in patients with OT VAs. In some patients, the site of origin may be intramural. Ablation of intramural OT VAs can be challenging to map and ablate due to deep intramural sites of origin. The coronary venous branches may permit mapping and ablation of intramural OT VAs.

Challenging anatomic and morphologic conditions of the left ventricular (LV) summit architecture and its surrounding sites may prevent sufficient heating of the targeted area during standard radiofrequency catheter ablation. Bipolar ablation can result in higher likelihood of efficacy for ablation of LV summit arrhythmias from inaccessible regions and increase the chance of achieving a transmural lesion. In this review, the authors describe the present approaches for bipolar ablation of the LV summit arrhythmias refractory to standard approaches.

Chemical ablation using the transcoronary arterial system has a lengthy but arduous history. Although it has shown to be efficacious in controlling ventricular arrhythmias, safety concerns from cannulation of the coronary arterial system to unwanted ethanol downstream effects have limited transcoronary ethanol ablation (TCEA)'s use. Retrograde coronary venous ethanol ablation (RCVEA) has shown promising results. Although it appears to be in its infancy, RCVEA appears to be the future of chemical ablation in comparison to TCEA due to its increased safety and efficacy. Prospective randomized trial data is needed for this adjunctive treatment to radiofrequency ablation.

Fluoroscopy use during catheter ablation (CA) of arrhythmias is associated with significant exposure to ionizing radiation and risk of orthopedic injuries. CA of ventricular arrhythmias (VAs) arising from the left ventricular (LV) summit requires vast knowledge of cardiac anatomy and careful imaging delineation of the different structures, which is frequently performed using fluoroscopy. Fluoroless CA procedures are feasible and appear to have similar safety and efficacy compared with conventional techniques. To be successfully performed, it is important to be fully acquainted with intracardiac echocardiography (ICE) imaging and electroanatomic mapping (EAM). We describe our approach for fluoroless LV summit CA.

The left ventricular summit (LVS) is the area in the highest portion of the left ventricular epicardium, bounded by the left coronary arteries and the coronary venous circulation, and can be surrounded by thick epicardial fat that may preclude epicardial ablation. Ablation of LVS ventricular arrhythmias (VA) can be achieved from adjacent structures with good success rates. The long-term freedom from LVS VA recurrence remains variable. This article reviews the spatial and anatomic relationship of the structures surrounding the LVS, which provide vantage points for ablation, and the acute and long-term outcomes of different ablation approaches in LVS VA ablation.

Video content accompanies this article at http://www.cardiacep.theclinics.com.

The left ventricular summit is a site of origin for idiopathic ventricular arrhythmias.
With advancements in mapping and ablation techniques, sites previously considered inaccessible can now be approached. Anatomical knowledge of the 3-dimen-
sional landmarks of this space is important, as critical structures reside within its
boundaries and are potentially liable to collateral injury during ablation. This article
reviews reported complications from ablation of ventricular arrhythmias arising
from the left ventricular summit and its vicinity and discusses the pros and cons
of different ablation technique and the role of an individualized anatomical approach
to reduce procedural related complications and improve outcomes.

CARDIAC ELECTROPHYSIOLOGY CLINICS

SERIES OF RELATED INTEREST

Cardiology Clinics
https://www.cardiology.theclinics.com/
Interventional Cardiology Clinics
https://www.interventional.theclinics.com/
Heart Failure Clinics
https://www.heartfailure.theclinics.com/

THE CLINICS ARE AVAILABLE ONLINE!
Access your subscription at:
www.theclinics.com

Foreword
Tubthumping

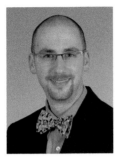 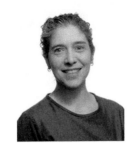

Jordan M. Prutkin, MD, MHS, FHRS   Emily P. Zeitler MD, MHS, FHRS

Consulting Editors

Years ago, we infrequently put an ablation catheter anywhere but the right ventricular outflow tract to ablate premature ventricular contractions (PVCs) or ventricular tachycardia in those with a normal heart. For patients with a cardiomyopathy, we'd do endocardial left ventricular or right ventricular ablation. In time, we started to feel comfortable ablating from most ventricular locations, even near the His bundle, finding ways to be successful and safe.

But there were times it felt like we were tubthumping the PVCs. They got knocked down, but they got up again. We needed better tools and techniques. The left ventricular summit has been an especially difficult place to be successful, but we learned how to ablate in the aortic root (watch out coronary ostia!), in the great cardiac vein (watch out coronary arteries!), in the interleaflet triangle below the left-right coronary cusps (get that catheter curve tight!), on the epicardial surface (let's try CO_2 insufflation for pericardial access!), or down the anterior interventricular vein (wire mapping!). Investigators have used alcohol ablation via septal perforators (he drinks a whiskey drink; he drinks a vodka drink!) and half normal saline (don't cry for me!). In addition to therapeutic improvements, our understanding of three-dimensional cardiac anatomy and our ability to localize ventricular arrhythmias using criteria based on the surface ECG improved. We can now more confidently discuss success and risks of the procedure with the patient and allow for better preprocedure planning. We could ablate from anywhere we could reach, and sometimes it was

okay to be close enough. Truth is, we thought it mattered that you be right on top of it, but does it? Bollocks. You might get lucky from where you could reach. And, hey, if one catheter couldn't get it done, maybe using two catheters for bipolar ablation would be successful.

That brings us to today and this latest issue of *Cardiac Electrophysiology Clinics*. Edited by Drs Pasquale Santangeli, Fermin Garcia, and Luis Sáenz, this issue on the left ventricular summit presents a wide overview of the anatomy of the summit, ventricular arrhythmias originating from the area, and how to ablate them. We thank the editors and authors for this excellent series of reviews. In time, our hope is that we will no longer be tubthumping PVCs, but we'll be singing, when we're winning!

Jordan M. Prutkin, MD, MHS, FHRS
Division of Cardiology
University of Washington
1959 NE Pacific Street, Box 356422
Seattle, WA 98195, USA

Emily P. Zeitler, MD, MHS, FHRS
Dartmouth Health and
The Dartmouth Institute
1 Medical Center Drive
Lebanon, NH, 03756, USA

E-mail addresses:
jprutkin@uw.edu (J.M. Prutkin)
emily.p.zeitler@hitchcock.org (E.P. Zeitler)

Card Electrophysiol Clin 15 (2023) xiii
https://doi.org/10.1016/j.ccep.2022.11.001
1877-9182/23/© 2022 Published by Elsevier Inc.

cardiacEP.theclinics.com

Preface

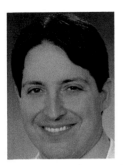 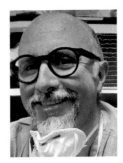 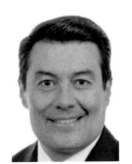

| Pasquale Santangeli, MD, PhD | Fermin C. Garcia, MD | Luis C. Sáenz, MD |
| | *Editors* | |

The left ventricular summit (LVS) is a common site of origin of ventricular arrhythmias (VAs) and undoubtedly represents one of the most challenging areas to map and effectively ablate VAs. Over the last several years, tremendous advancements have been made in the understanding of the anatomic relationships between the LVS and other adjacent vantage points within the right and left ventricular outflow tracts; this has facilitated a more streamlined mapping approach and more effective ablation strategies.

This issue of the *Cardiac Electrophysiology Clinics* is entirely focused on the LVS as a source of VAs. The anatomy of the region, the relationships with adjacent structures, and the different approaches for mapping and ablation are reviewed by international leaders in the field. We are pleased to present this work to the readers and wish to thank all the authors for their outstanding contributions.

Pasquale Santangeli, MD, PhD
Section of Cardiac Electrophysiology
Cleveland Clinic
Cleveland, OH, USA

Fermin C. Garcia, MD
Section of Cardiac Electrophysiology
Hospital of the University of Pennsylvania
Philadelphia, PA, USA

Luis C. Sáenz, MD
Internacional Arrhythmia Center
Fundación Cardio Infantil-Instituto de Cardiología
Bogotá, Colombia

E-mail addresses:
Pasquale.Santangeli@uphs.upenn.edu
pasquale.santangeli@gmail.com (P. Santangeli)
Fermin.Garcia@pennmedicine.upenn.edu
(F.C. Garcia)
luchossaenzmorales@yahoo.com (L.C. Sáenz)

Card Electrophysiol Clin 15 (2023) xv
https://doi.org/10.1016/j.ccep.2022.10.005
1877-9182/23/© 2022 Published by Elsevier Inc.

Revisiting the Anatomy of the Left Ventricular Summit

Shumpei Mori, MD, PhD[a,b,*], Justin Hayase, MD[a,b],
Aadhavi Sridharan, MD, PhD[a,b], Koji Fukuzawa, MD, PhD[c],
Kalyanam Shivkumar, MD, PhD[a,b], Jason S. Bradfield, MD[a,b]

KEYWORDS

- Cardiac anatomy • Epicardial ablation • Intracardiac echocardiography • Left ventricular summit

KEY POINTS

- The summit of the left ventricle was introduced by Wallace A. McAlpine as the highest region in the left ventricular muscle.
- The left ventricular summit corresponds to the epicardial part of the basal superior free wall, extending from the base of the left coronary aortic sinus.
- The left ventricular summit is surrounded by the infundibulum, pulmonary root, left coronary aortic sinus, left atrial appendage, and coronary vessels.

INTRODUCTION

The left ventricular summit was first introduced by Wallace A. McAlpine as the literally highest region of the left ventricular muscle (**Fig. 1**), when the heart is sat in a physiologic position within the thoracic cavity.[1] This anatomic concept of the left ventricular summit was introduced to the field of electrophysiology in relation to the ventricular arrhythmias originating from these specific regions.[2,3] Numerous works focusing around this specific region have been published.[4–19] However, the anatomy of the left ventricular summit is complicated, with many important surrounding structures. Thus, multiple anatomic images are required to help with comprehensive understanding of the region. Without a precise appreciation of the anatomy of the left ventricular summit, ventricular arrhythmias originating from the region cannot be characterized and optimal strategy for mapping and ablation cannot be selected. Therefore, we revisit the anatomy of the left ventricular summit by demonstrating multiple anatomic images, including original images from Wallace A. McAlpine Collection.

CONCEPT OF THE LEFT VENTRICULAR SUMMIT

McAlpine, in his original textbook,[1] indicated the left ventricular summit as the highest region of the left ventricular muscle, when the heart is placed in attitudinal orientation. When his concept was introduced to the field of electrophysiology, left ventricular summit was subsequently referred to as the fan-shaped epicardial region extending from the base of the left coronary aortic sinus toward the basal superior free wall of the left ventricle,

Funding: This work was made possible by support from NIH grants OT2OD023848 to K. Shivkumar.
[a] UCLA Cardiac Arrhythmia Center, UCLA Health System, David Geffen School of Medicine at UCLA, Los Angeles, CA, USA; [b] UCLA Cardiovascular Interventional Programs, Department of Medicine, David Geffen School of Medicine at UCLA & UCLA Health System, Los Angeles, CA, USA; [c] Section of Arrhythmia, Division of Cardiovascular Medicine, Department of Internal Medicine, Kobe University Graduate School of Medicine
* Corresponding author. UCLA Cardiac Arrhythmia Center, UCLA Health System, David Geffen School of Medicine at UCLA, 650 Charles E. Young Dr. South, Center of the Health Science, Suite #46-119C, Los Angeles, CA 90095.
E-mail address: shumpei@g.ucla.edu

Card Electrophysiol Clin 15 (2023) 1–8
https://doi.org/10.1016/j.ccep.2022.04.003
1877-9182/23/© 2022 Elsevier Inc. All rights reserved.

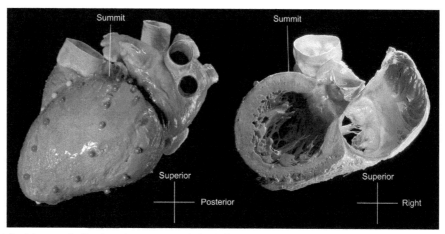

Fig. 1. Original images indicating the summit of the left ventricle. McAlpine indicates the summit of the left ventricle as a confined region located at the highest part of the left ventricular muscle, when the heart is placed in a physiologic fashion. (*Illustration courtesy* UCLA Cardiac Arrhythmia Center, Wallace A. McAlpine MD Collection; reproduced with permission.)

demarcated by the left anterior descending artery antero-medially and by the left circumflex artery postero-laterally (**Fig. 2**). In the field of echocardiography, this region should be the basal superior (commonly referred to as anterior) region of the left ventricle. Thus, the left ventricular summit is located at the corner between the anterior interventricular groove and left atrioventricular groove.

RELATIONSHIP WITH THE CORONARY VESSELS

Antero-medial part of the summit is related to the left anterior descending artery and anterior interventricular vein, and postero-lateral part of the summit is related to the left circumflex artery and great cardiac vein. Regarding the arterial supply, in addition to the left anterior descending artery and left circumflex artery demarcating the summit, the diagonal branch, high-lateral branch, and obtuse marginal branch can run on the left ventricular summit (see **Fig. 2**). Coronary venous anatomy demonstrates wide variation,[1,10,19] in terms of the topographic relationships between the anterior interventricular vein-great cardiac vein junction and the aortic root, between the anterior interventricular vein and left anterior descending artery, and between the great cardiac vein and left circumflex artery. As the coronary vessels are buried in the epicardial adipose tissue, the vertical distance from coronary venous tributaries to the left ventricular summit is also highly variable (**Fig. 3**).

AORTOMITRAL CONTINUITY

The left fibrous trigone is a thick fibrous tissue supporting the bottom of the left coronary aortic sinus.

It supports the lateral side of the anterior mitral leaflet. Thus, the left fibrous trigone is related to the location of the supero-lateral commissure of the mitral valve (**Fig. 4**). The left fibrous trigone is generally covered by left ventricular myocardium, creating the characteristic angle between the aortic orifice and mitral valve orifice. This angulation at the bottom of the left coronary aortic sinus is referred to as the left ostial process,[1] which is the most basal and medial part of the left ventricular summit (see **Fig. 4**). This left ostial process corresponds to the so-called aortomitral continuity, confusingly used in the field of electrophysiology.[2,4,6,7] In the strict anatomic sense, the aortomitral continuity is the region between the anterior mitral leaflet and the interleaflet triangle between the left and noncoronary aortic sinuses, which is generally devoid of any ventricular myocardium.[20,21]

STRUCTURES SURROUNDING THE LEFT VENTRICULAR SUMMIT

The left ventricular summit is surrounded by the aortic root medially, left atrial appendage postero-laterally, infundibulum and pulmonary root anteriorly, and pulmonary trunk superiorly. This compartment-like space was referred to as the left coronary fossa by McAlpine.[1] Thus, the left ventricular summit composes the floor of this compartment. Careful appreciation of each sectional image obtained by progressive virtual dissection of the volume-rendered images around the left ventricular summit is the best way to understand three-dimensional complexity of this region (**Figs. 5** and **6**). Specifically, the anterior wall of this compartment is not composed of the

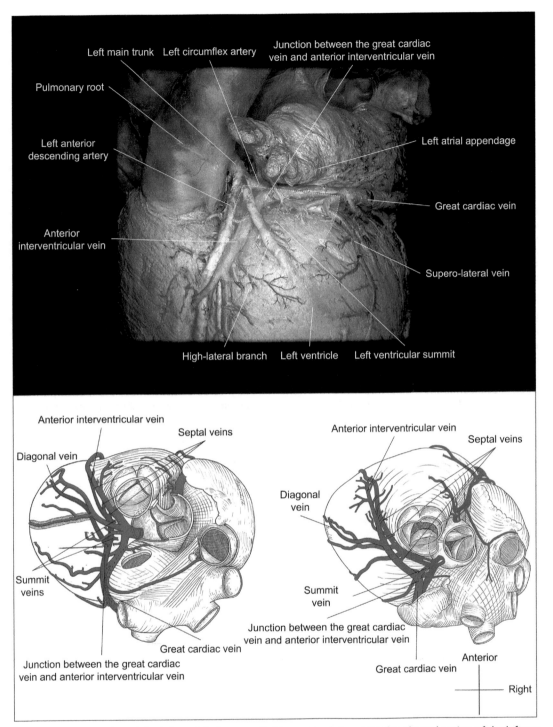

Fig. 2. Coronary vessels and the left ventricular summit. Upper panel shows the fan-shaped region of the left ventricular summit (*yellow*) in relation to the pulmonary root, left atrial appendage, and coronary vessels. Lower panels show the multiple coronary venous tributaries distributing to the left ventricular summit and ventricular septum. (*Illustration courtesy* UCLA Cardiac Arrhythmia Center, Wallace A. McAlpine MD Collection; reproduced with permission.)

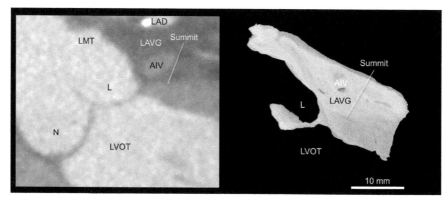

Fig. 3. Frontal section of the left ventricular summit. Left panel is the multiplanar reconstruction image of the cardiac computed tomography, and the right panel is the comparable gross dissection sample of the left ventricular summit. Left ventricular summit supports the left coronary aortic sinus (*L*), exhibiting a bird beak-shape appearance. Thick epicardial adipose tissue of the left atrioventricular groove (LAVG) and variation in the location of the anterior interventricular vein (AIV) in relation to the summit can be appreciated. LAD, left anterior descending artery; LMT, left main trunk; LVOT, left ventricular outflow tract; N, noncoronary aortic sinus.

pulmonary root but of the elevated infundibulum, also referred to as the posterior free wall of the right ventricular outflow tract (see **Fig. 4**). This is one of the risky regions of perforation during any invasive approach to the right ventricular outflow tract, in addition to the medial free wall of the right ventricular outflow tract (see **Fig. 4**). The medial wall of this compartment is the left coronary aortic sinus. Thus, at the most proximal part of the fan-shaped left ventricular summit, the left ventricular free wall directly supports the anterior half of the

left coronary aortic sinus (see **Figs. 4–6**). Generally, left ventricular summit visualized in left ventricular basal short-axis section exhibits a bird beak-shape appearance (see **Fig. 3**), showing the thin free wall (<3.0 mm) supporting the left coronary aortic sinus.[22] Thus, the medial part of the summit can be approached via the left coronary aortic sinus. In other words, a ventricular arrhythmia that can be ablated from the left coronary aortic sinus can be deemed as an arrhythmia originating from the medial margin of the left

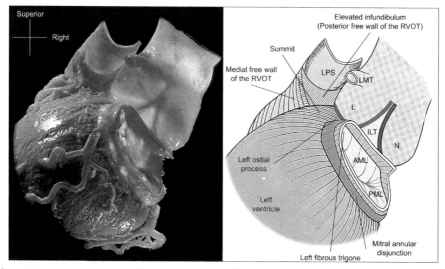

Fig. 4. Left ventricular summit viewed from the posterior direction. These images beautifully show the elevated infundibulum as the wall anterior to the summit and the left ostial process as the most postero-medial part of the summit. Left ventricular summit supports the anterior base of the left coronary aortic sinus (*L*). AML, anterior mitral leaflet; ILT, interleaflet triangle; LMT, left main trunk; LPS, left-adjacent pulmonary sinus; N, noncoronary aortic sinus; PML, posterior mitral leaflet; RVOT, right ventricular outflow tract. (*Illustration courtesy* UCLA Cardiac Arrhythmia Center, Wallace A. McAlpine MD Collection; reproduced with permission.)

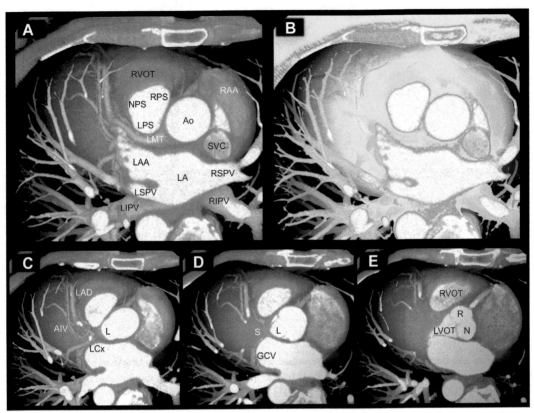

Fig. 5. Progressive dissection of the left ventricular summit from the superior direction. From panel (*A*) to panel (*E*), parallel plane-cut from the superior direction is applied. Panels A and B are in the same section. In real settings, coronary vessels visualized in panel A are buried in the thick epicardial adipose tissue (*B*). Relationships between the summit (*S*), aortic root, left atrial appendage (LAA), and right ventricular outflow tract (RVOT) and pulmonary root can be appreciated. AIV, anterior interventricular vein; Ao, ascending aorta; GCV, great cardiac vein; L, left coronary aortic sinus; LA, left atrium; LAD, left anterior descending artery; LCx, left circumflex artery; LIPV, left inferior pulmonary vein; LMT, left main trunk; LPS, left adjacent pulmonary sinus; LSPV, left superior pulmonary vein; LVOT, left ventricular outflow tract; N, noncoronary aortic sinus; NPS, nonadjacent pulmonary sinus; R, right coronary aortic sinus; RAA, right atrial appendage; RIPV, right inferior pulmonary vein; RSPV, right superior pulmonary vein; RPS, right adjacent pulmonary sinus; SVC, superior vena cava.

ventricular summit. The postero-lateral part of the compartment is covered by the left atrial appendage (see **Figs. 1** and **5**), suggesting the feasibility of the approach via the inferior wall of the left atrial appendage,[11] although the thick epicardial fat of the left atrioventricular groove prevents the effective energy delivery. The endocardial side of the left ventricular summit corresponds to the area adjacent to the supero-lateral commissure of the mitral valve, located at 12 o'clock of the mitral annulus (see **Figs. 4** and **6**).

INTRACARDIAC ECHOCARDIOGRAPHY OF THE LEFT VENTRICULAR SUMMIT

The left ventricular summit is an epicardial region, and there is thick epicardial adipose tissue of the atrioventricular groove that limits the image quality

around the summit. Thus, the clinical utility of the intracardiac echocardiography during catheter ablation of the left ventricular summit is controversial. Even the thickness of the myocardium at the summit, as well as the coronary vessels, are not always clearly discerned. However, when using alternative endocardial approaches, intracardiac echocardiography is useful to detect the left coronary aortic sinus, interleaflet triangle between the right and left coronary aortic sinuses, anterior mitral leaflet, and right and left ventricular outflow tract. Conventional views from the right atrial appendage can demonstrate an image identical to the coronal section involving the summit, inferior pyramidal space, and infero-septal process[23] (**Fig. 7**). When reading the intracardiac echocardiographic image or comparing it with other imaging modalities, it is important to rotate the image to

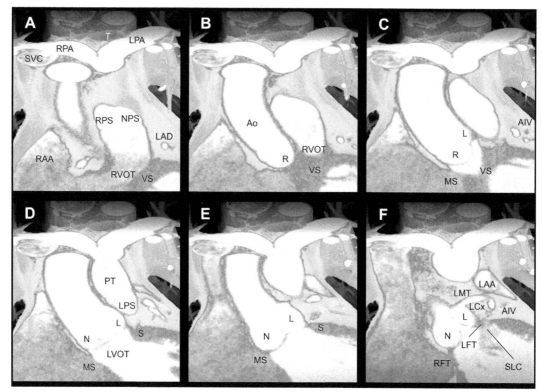

Fig. 6. Progressive virtual dissection of the left ventricular summit from the anterior direction. The heart is viewed from the cranial 25° direction. Basal superior part of the ventricular septum (VS) tilts toward left and posterior direction (*A*). From the panel A to panel F, the parallel plane-cut from the anterior direction is applied. The posterior free wall of the right ventricular outflow tract (RVOT) gets apart from the ventricular septum (*B, C*) anterior to the left ventricular summit (S). Left ventricular summit mainly supports the left coronary aortic sinus (L) (*D, E*). At the most posterior part, left ventricular summit is adjacent to the left fibrous trigone (LFT) and supero-lateral commissure (SLC) of the mitral valve (*F*). AIV, anterior interventricular vein; Ao, ascending aorta; LAA, left atrial appendage; LAD, left anterior descending artery; LCx, left circumflex artery; LMT, left main trunk; LPA, left pulmonary artery; LPS, left adjacent pulmonary sinus; LVOT, left ventricular outflow tract; MS, membranous septum; N, noncoronary aortic sinus; NPS, nonadjacent pulmonary sinus; PT, pulmonary trunk; R, right coronary aortic sinus; RAA, right atrial appendage; RFT, right fibrous trigone; RPA, right pulmonary artery; RPS, right adjacent pulmonary sinus; SVC, superior vena cava; T, trachea.

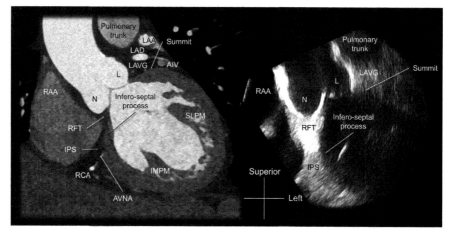

Fig. 7. Intracardiac echocardiographic images of the left ventricular summit. Right panel is the intracardiac echocardiographic image viewed from the right atrial appendage (RAA) with comparable computed tomographic coronal section image (*left panel*). The ablation catheter is placed at the infero-septal process. AIV, anterior interventricular vein; AVNA, atrioventricular nodal artery; IMPM, infero-medial papillary muscle; IPS, inferior pyramidal space; L, left coronary aortic sinus; LAA, left atrial appendage; LAD, left anterior descending artery; LAVG, left atrioventricular groove; N, noncoronary aortic sinus; RCA, right coronary artery; RFT, right fibrous trigone; SLPM, supero-lateral papillary muscle.

achieve physiologic orientation. Such rotation helps one understand the complicated anatomy visualized in each image far easier than placing the probe always at the top of the monitor.[24]

SUMMARY

The anatomy of the left ventricular summit has been revisited. Precise anatomic appreciation of this complicated region in relation to the surrounding structures will help make correct diagnoses, consider appropriate treatments, and avoid complications.

CLINICS CARE POINTS

- The anatomy of the left ventricular summit is complicated, with many important surrounding structures, including the infundibulum, pulmonary root, left coronary aortic sinus, interleaflet triangle, left atrial appendage, and coronary vessels.
- As these anatomical structures also show individual variation, precise evaluation of the three-dimensional anatomy in each case with multiple imaging modalities would be fundamental for successful elimination of the arrhythmia originating from the left ventricular summit.

DISCLOSURE

The authors have nothing to disclose.

REFERENCES

1. McAlpine WA. Heart and coronary arteries: an anatomical atlas for clinical diagnosis, radiological investigation, and surgical treatment. New York: Springer-Verlag; 1975.
2. Yamada T, Litovsky SH, Kay GN. The left ventricular ostium: an anatomic concept relevant to idiopathic ventricular arrhythmias. Circ Arrhythm Electrophysiol 2008;1:396–404.
3. Steven D, Roberts-Thomson KC, Seiler J, et al. Ventricular tachycardia arising from the aortomitral continuity in structural heart disease: characteristics and therapeutic considerations for an anatomically challenging area of origin. Circ Arrhythm Electrophysiol 2009;2:660–6.
4. Yamada T, McElderry HT, Dipalladium H, et al. Idiopathic ventricular arrhythmias originating from the left ventricular summit: anatomic concepts relevant to ablation. Circ AR Rhythm Electrophysiol 2010;3:616–23.
5. Yokokawa M, Good E, Chugh A, et al. Intramural idiopathic ventricular arrhythmias originating in the intraventricular septum: mapping and ablation. Circ Arrhythm Electrophysiol 2012;5:258–63.
6. Kumagai K. Idiopathic ventricular arrhythmias arising from the left ventricular outflow tract: Tips and tricks. J Arrhythm 2014;30:221–31.
7. Lerman BB. Mechanism, diagnosis, and treatment of outflow tract tachycardia. Nat Rev Cardiol 2015; 12:597–608.
8. Baldinger SH, Kumar S, Barbhaiya CR, et al. Epicardial radiofrequency ablation Failure during ablation Procedures for ventricular arrhythmias: Reasons and implications for Outcomes. Circ Arrhythm Electrophysiol 2015;8:1422–32.
9. Kreidieh B, Rodríguez-Mañero M, Schurmann P, et al. Retrograde coronary venous ethanol infusion for ablation of refractory ventricular tachycardia. Circ Arrhythm Electrophysiol 2016;9:e004352.
10. Komatsu Y, Nogami A, Shinoda Y, et al. Idiopathic ventricular arrhythmias originating from the vicinity of the communicating vein of cardiac venous Systems at the left ventricular summit. Circ Arrhythm Electrophysiol 2018;11:e005386.
11. Yakubov A, Salayev O, Hamrayev R, et al. A case of successful ablation of ventricular tachycardia focus in the left ventricular summit through the left atrial appendage: a case report. Eur Heart J Case Rep 2018;2:yty110.
12. Romero J, Diaz JC, Hayase J, et al. Intramyocardial radiofrequency ablation of ventricular arrhythmias using intracoronary wire mapping and a coronary reentry system: Description of a novel technique. Heartrhythm Case Rep 2018;4:285–92.
13. Enriquez A, Baranchuk A, Briceno D, et al. How to use the 12-lead ECG to predict the site of origin of idiopathic ventricular arrhythmias. Heart Rhythm 2019;16:1538–44.
14. Cheung JW, Anderson RH, Markowitz SM, et al. Catheter ablation of arrhythmias originating from the left ventricular outflow tract. JACC Clin Electrophysiol 2019;5:1–12.
15. Kodali S, Santangeli P, Garcia FC. Mapping and ablation of arrhythmias from Uncommon Sites (aortic Cusp, pulmonary artery, and left ventricular summit). Card Electrophysiol Clin 2019;11:665–74.
16. Anderson RD, Kumar S, Parameswaran R, et al. Differentiating right- and left-Sided outflow tract ventricular arrhythmias: classical ECG signatures and prediction algorithms. Circ Arrhythm Electrophysiol 2019;12:e007392.
17. Briceño DF, Enriquez A, Liang JJ, et al. Septal coronary venous mapping to Guide Substrate Characterization and ablation of Intramural septal ventricular arrhythmia. JACC Clin Electrophysiol 2019;5:789–800.
18. Bradfield JS. Redefining optimal targets for intramural ventricular arrhythmias: planning for combat! JACC Clin Electrophysiol 2020;6:1349–52.
19. Tavares L, Fuentes S, Lador A, et al. Venous anatomy of the left ventricular summit: therapeutic

implications for ethanol infusion. Heart Rhythm 2021; 18(9):1557–65.

20. Mori S, Fukuzawa K, Takaya T, et al. Clinical cardiac structural anatomy reconstructed within the cardiac contour using multidetector-row computed tomography: left ventricular outflow tract. Clin Anat 2016;29: 353–63.

21. Mori S, Tretter JT, Spicer DE, et al. What is the real cardiac anatomy? Clin Anat 2019;32:288–309.

22. Toh H, Mori S, Tretter JT, et al. Living anatomy of the ventricular myocardial Crescents supporting the coronary aortic sinuses. Semin Thoric Cardiovasc Surg 2020;32:230–41.

23. Li A, Zuberi Z, Bradfield JS, et al. Endocardial ablation of ventricular ectopic beats arising from the basal inferoseptal process of the left ventricle. Heart Rhythm 2018;15:1356–62.

24. Khakpour H, Mori S, Bradfield JS, et al. How to use intracardiac echocardiography to recognize normal cardiac anatomy. Card Electrophysiol Clin 2021;13: 273–83.

Deductive Electrocardiographic Analysis of Left Ventricular Summit Arrhythmias

Matthew G. Hanson, MD, Andres Enriquez, MD*

KEYWORDS

• ECG analysis • LVS PVC • LVS VT

KEY POINTS

- The LVS ECG is characterized by either a RBBB pattern or LBBB pattern with early transition (V2 or V3), taller R wave in III than II, more negative Q wave in aVL than aVR, and often a pseudo-delta wave (or maximum deflection index > 0.55).
- A V2 pattern break (abrupt loss of R wave in V2 versus V1 and V3) suggests an anatomic origin close to the anterior interventricular groove and is characteristic of arrhythmias from the LVS or adjacent endocardial structures.
- A RBBB morphology without transition is the most common pattern of arrhythmias from the accessible region. Features that suggest an origin from the inaccessible region include a smaller R/S ratio in V1, R-wave amplitude ratio in lead III/II and Q-wave amplitude ratio in aVL/aVR.

BACKGROUND

Despite the advances of intracardiac mapping, the 12-lead electrocardiogram (ECG) remains the initial and simplest mapping tool at clinicians' disposal for localization of ventricular arrhythmias (VAs).

When catheter ablation is being considered, the ECG is helpful to predict the site of arrhythmia origin and eventually the most likely site of arrythmia elimination. Although in most focal VAs both sites are identical, this is not always the case, and this differentiation may be particularly important in left ventricular (LV) summit arrhythmias. The site of origin, which is defined as the site of earliest electrical activation, corresponds to the epicardial aspect of the LV ostium. Conversely, arrhythmia elimination in these cases is rarely achieved from the epicardial surface and most often requires ablation from one or multiple adjacent endocardial sites.

Interpretation of the ECG requires an attitudinal approach,[1] which involves understanding cardiac anatomy and the relationship between different structures as they are naturally situated within the chest. In the present article, we review the ECG patterns that suggest an LV summit origin and the clues that point toward the site of successful ablation.

ANATOMIC CONSIDERATIONS

As described by McAlpine, the LV summit is located at the high point of the LV epicardium, adjacent to the bifurcation of the left main coronary artery (LMCA)[2,3] (**Fig. 1**). It is a fan-shaped space defined medially by the left anterior descending (LAD) artery and laterally by the left circumflex artery, and lies superiorly to the aortic portion of the LV ostium and the anterior interventricular sulcus.[1] The base LV summit occurs at the level of the first

Division of Cardiology, Queen's University, Kingston, Ontario, Canada
* Corresponding author. Division of Cardiology, Queen's University, 76 Stuart Street, Kingston, Ontario K7L 2V7, Canada.
E-mail address: Andres.Enriquez@kingstonhsc.ca

Card Electrophysiol Clin 15 (2023) 9–14
https://doi.org/10.1016/j.ccep.2022.04.004
1877-9182/23/© 2022 Elsevier Inc. All rights reserved.

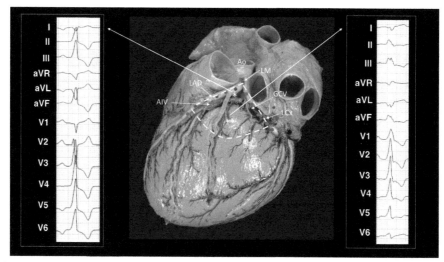

Fig. 1. *Left ventricular summit anatomic landmarks and ECG patterns.* Ventricular arrhythmias from the antero-medial aspect (inaccessible region) are characterized by an LBBB morphology with V2 or V3 transition, whereas those from the postero-lateral aspect (accessible region) exhibit an RBBB morphology with no transition. A smaller R/S ratio in V1, R-wave amplitude ratio in lead III/II (<1.13) and Q-wave amplitude ratio in aVL/aVR (<1.45) are features that suggest an origin from the inaccessible region. *Abbreviations:* **, accessible region; *, inaccessible region; Ao, Aorta, LM, left main; GCV, great coronary vein; LAD, left anterior descending artery; LCx, left circumflex artery; AIV, anterior interventricular vein. (Illustration courtesy UCLA Cardiac Arrhythmia Center, Wallace A. McAlpine MD collection).

septal perforator with an imaginary line traced over the LV epicardium.[4]

The LV summit is bisected by the great cardiac vein (GCV) into an anterior and medial portion (the inaccessible region) and a more posterior and lateral portion (the accessible region).[5] This anatomic division is useful from a practical perspective. Thus, arrhythmias from the postero-lateral summit can often be eliminated by ablation from the coronary venous system or eventually via percutaneous epicardial approach. Conversely, the antero-medial aspect is largely inaccessible to epicardial ablation due to proximity to the coronary arteries (LAD, LMCA) and overlying epicardial fat. VAs from the inaccessible region need to be targeted from endocardial vantage points such as the left coronary cusp (LCC) or right/left cusp junction,[6–8] the endocardial LV outflow tract (LVOT),[9] the septal right ventricular outflow tract,[6,10] or the left pulmonary cusp.[11]

GENERAL ELECTROCARDIOGRAPHIC FEATURES

With the anatomy of the LV ostium in mind, we can apply some deductive reasoning to a surface ECG and aid in localization of particular VAs. It is important to keep in mind that these determinations can be affected by individual anatomic variation, body habitus, and lead placement.

Frontal Plane Axis

Vertical dimension (superior/inferior axis)
Anatomically, the LV summit is at the superior portion of the LV. Therefore, any ectopic arrhythmia generated from this area will depolarize the heart in a cranial to caudal direction, generating an inferiorly directed QRS axis with positive deflections (monophasic R waves) in leads II and III.[1]

Horizontal dimension (right/left axis)
LV summit arrhythmias typically have a right axis, consistent with its origin on the left side of the midline. Lead I is predominantly negative, sometimes exhibiting a QS pattern. In addition, lead III is more positive than lead II and lead aVL is more negative than aVR, all of which reflect left-to-right depolarization forces.[6,9,12,13]

Bundle Branch Block Pattern

LV summit arrhythmias may exhibit a left bundle branch block (LBBB) or right bundle branch block (RBBB) morphology, depending on their more medial or lateral origin within the region. Thus, an RBBB pattern is observed in virtually all arrhythmias from the accessible area, but is rare in those with an origin in the inaccessible area, which are usually characterized by an LBBB pattern (see **Fig. 1**).[9,12] A large multicenter series including 238 patients with ventricular tachycardia (VT) and/or premature ventricular complexes (PVCs) originating from the LV summit showed that an LBBB is the more prevalent pattern, accounting for 60% of all cases.[14]

Precordial Transition and "Pattern Breaks"

As a general principle, precordial transition becomes progressively earlier as the site of origin moves from the septum to the more lateral aspect of the LV summit. VAs from the lateral LV summit usually have no precordial transition, exhibiting a monomorphic R wave in V_1 and positive concordance across the precordial leads (all positive precordial leads), whereas VAs from the more septal aspect present an LBBB with V_2 or V_3 precordial transition (rarely V_4).[9] A Q-wave in V_1 is associated with a lower rate of ablation success because it indicates a medial/septal origin, which is generally within the inaccessible region.[12]

Some VAs with LBBB morphology may exhibit a "V_2 pattern break," which is a loss of R-wave in V_2 when compared with V_1 and V_3. This suggests that the depolarization is arising from the septal LV summit, which is anatomically opposite to lead V_2 near the interventricular sulcus lying close to the LAD (**Fig. 2**). This has been further described as abrupt R-wave transition in lead V_3 (ATV3; see later), which can exist independent of the pattern break and also suggests an origin from the septal margin of the LV summit.[7]

QRS Duration and Pseudo-delta Wave

As we have described, the LV summit is an epicardial region of the heart. Depolarization of the ventricle from epicardial structures generate QRS complexes with slurring of the initial deflection of the QRS, also known as a pseudo-delta wave. This slow initial depolarization is caused by slow cell-to-cell conduction of the electrical impulse until it can access the more rapid depolarization of the Purkinje system. We can view this initial delay in multiple ways on surface ECG, as follows (**Fig. 3**)[2,15,16]:

1. Pseudo-delta wave $\geq$ 34 ms.
2. Intrinsicoid deflection time in V2 (interval from the earliest ventricular activation to the peak of the R wave in V2) $\geq$ 85 ms.
3. Maximum deflection index (MDI) (shortest interval to maximum positive or negative deflection in precordial leads divided by total QRS duration) $\geq$ 0.55..
4. Shortest RS complex, $\geq$ 121 ms.

DIFFERENTIAL DIAGNOSIS

Differential diagnosis of LV summit arrhythmias includes arrhythmias from neighboring endocardial sites such as the LCC and aortomitral continuity in case of RBBB pattern or the right–left cusp commissure in case of LBBB pattern (**Fig. 4**). Differentiation is not always easy due to significant

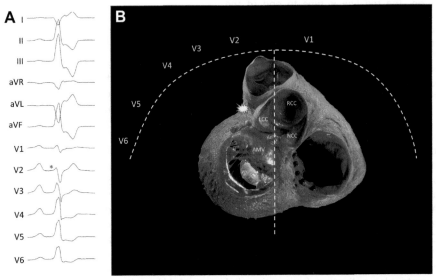

Fig. 2. *V2 pattern break in LV summit PVC.* The ECG demonstrates an LBBB pattern with right inferior axis and V3 transition. Note the loss of R-wave in V_2 when compared with V_1 and V_3. This finding reflects depolarization from the interventricular sulcus near the LAD, which is anatomically opposite lead V_2. *Abbreviations:* AMV, anterior mitral valve; LCC, left coronary cusp; NCC, noncoronary cusp; RCC, right coronary cusp. (Illustration courtesy UCLA Cardiac Arrhythmia Center, Wallace A. McAlpine MD collection).

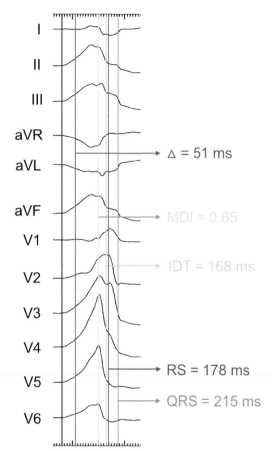

I

II

III

aVR

aVL Δ = 51 ms

aVF   MDI = 0.65

V1

V2   IDT = 168 ms

V3

V4

V5   RS = 178 ms

            QRS = 215 ms

V6

Fig. 3. *Example of LV summit PVC with markers for common ECG findings consistent with an epicardial focus.* The black line represents the onset of epicardial depolarization. The red line is time to end of the pseudo-delta wave (Δ) (epicardial $\geq$ 34 ms). The orange line is the maximum deflection index (calculated as shortest interval to maximum deflection in precordial leads/total QRS duration; epicardial $\geq$ 0.55). The green line represents the intrinsicoid deflection time in V_2 (epicardial $\geq$ 85 ms). The purple line represents the shortest RS interval (epicardial $\geq$ 121 ms).

overlap between these closely related structures, with the possibility of preferential conduction and potential for multiple exit sites.[17]

A QS pattern in lead I is more often seen in LV summit arrhythmias, whereas most endocardial LVOT VAs exhibit an rS pattern in lead I.[6,13] Additionally, the MDI is higher in epicardial VAs (0.52 vs 0.45; *P* .0005) and both the III/II and aVL/aVR ratios are greater than in those from endocardial LVOT structures.[13] The latter because ventricular activation from epicardial foci propagates toward the LV lateral wall before activating the His Bundle region, therefore resulting in a decrease in the amplitude of an R wave in lead II and Q wave in lead aVR

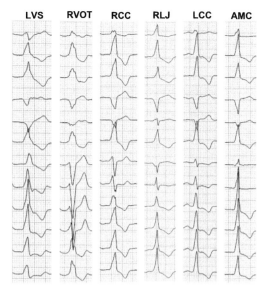

LVS   RVOT   RCC   RLJ   LCC   AMC

Fig. 4. *Twelve-lead ECG of LV summit PVC and comparison to endocardial sites within the outflow tract.* Note typical ECG from the accessible region, characterized by RBBB pattern, right inferior axis, R-wave amplitude in III higher than II, and lead aVL more negative than aVR. Abbreviations: AMC, aortomitral continuity; LBBB, left bundle branch block; LCC, left coronary cusp; LVS, left ventricular summit; RBBB, right bundle branch block; RCC, right coronary cusp; RLJ, right-left cusp junction; RVOT, right ventricle outflow tract.

and an increase in the amplitude of an R wave in lead III.

ELECTROCARDIOGRAPHIC PREDICTORS OF SUCCESSFUL ABLATION SITE

Certain ECG features may point toward the most likely site of successful ablation. Jauregui Abularach and colleagues[8] studied a group of 16 consecutive patients with VT/PVCs mapped to the distal GCV/proximal anterior interventricular vein (AIV). In all these cases, an initial ablation attempt was undertaken from the LCC and/or adjacent LV endocardium, followed by ablation from the coronary venous system or epicardium if coronary angiography showed a safe distance (>10 mm) to the left coronary artery. The authors found that a smaller Q-wave amplitude ratio in aVL/aVR (<1.45) and R-wave amplitude ratio in lead III/II (<1.13) were associated with successful ablation from the LCC or adjacent LV endocardium (*P* .043 for both). This group also exhibited a shorter anatomic distance between the earliest GCV/AIV site and the closes endocardial site (11.0 $\pm$ 6.5 vs 20.4 $\pm$ 12.1 mm; *P* .048).

Recently, Liao *and colleagues*[7] reported a novel ECG pattern characterized by LBBB with an ATV3 defined as an R-wave amplitude in lead V3 three times greater than that in V2. Among outflow tract PVCs with an epicardial or intramural origin (n = 12), the ATV3 pattern predicted successful ablation from the interleaflet triangle between the LCC and right coronary cusp in 75% of cases (sensitivity of 55% and specificity of 92%).

When ablation from the coronary venous system and adjacent LV/RV endocardial sites fails, the ECG may help identify suitable candidates for percutaneous epicardial ablation.[12] Santangeli *and colleagues*[12] reported that 3 ECG features were more prevalent in successful versus unsuccessful cases: Q-wave amplitude ratio in aVL/aVR greater than 1.85, R/S ratio of greater than 2 in V_1, and absence of q waves in lead V_1. All these indexes reflect a more lateral site of origin, away from the midline and the apex of the LV summit triangle. In this study, the presence of at least 2 of the 3 ECG criteria was associated with successful epicardial ablation with a 100% sensitivity and 72% specificity.

SUMMARY

The surface ECG allows the clinician to suspect when VT/PVCs likely originate in the LV summit, which is helpful for preprocedural planning. Features such as the bundle branch block pattern, R ratio in lead III/II and Q ratio in lead aVL/aVR suggest a more medial or lateral origin and help to predict whether successful ablation can be achieved from the coronary venous system or alternatively from adjacent endocardial vantage points.

FUNDING

None.

REFERENCES

1. Enriquez A, Baranchuk A, Briceno D, et al. How to use the 12-lead ECG to predict the site of origin of idiopathic ventricular arrhythmias. Heart Rhythm 2019;16(10):1538–44. https://doi.org/10.1016/j.hrthm.2019.04.002. Available at:.
2. Enriquez A, Malavassi F, Saenz LC, et al. How to map and ablate left ventricular summit arrhythmias. Heart Rhythm 2017;14(1):141–8. https://doi.org/10.1016/j.hrthm.2016.09.018. Available at:.
3. Am Heart J [Internet]. 1976;92(4):545Heart and coronary arteries: by wallace A. McAlpine, M.D. New York: Springer-Verlag; 1975. p. 223. Available at: https://www.sciencedirect.com/science/article/pii/S0002870376800646.
4. Kuniewicz M, Baszko A, Ali D, et al. Left ventricular summit—concept, anatomical structure and clinical significance. Diagnostics 2021;11(8):1–14.
5. Tzeis S, Asvestas D, Yen Ho S, et al. Electrocardiographic landmarks of idiopathic ventricular arrhythmia origins. Heart 2019;105(14):1109–16.
6. Komatsu Y, Nogami A, Shinoda Y, et al. Idiopathic ventricular arrhythmias originating from the vicinity of the communicating vein of cardiac venous systems at the left ventricular summit. Circ Arrhythm Electrophysiol 2018;11(1):1–10.
7. Liao H, Wei W, Tanager KS, et al. Left ventricular summit arrhythmias with an abrupt V3 transition: anatomy of the aortic interleaflet triangle vantage point. Heart Rhythm 2021;18(1):10–9. https://doi.org/10.1016/j.hrthm.2020.07.021. Available at:.
8. Jauregui Abularach ME, Campos B, Park KM, et al. Ablation of ventricular arrhythmias arising near the anterior epicardial veins from the left sinus of Valsalva region: ECG features, anatomic distance, and outcome. Heart Rhythm [Internet] 2012;9(6):865–73. https://doi.org/10.1016/j.hrthm.2012.01.022. Available at:.
9. Yamada T, Kumar V, Yoshida N, et al. Eccentric activation patterns in the left ventricular outflow tract during idiopathic ventricular arrhythmias originating from the left ventricular summit: a pitfall for predicting the sites of ventricular arrhythmia origins. Circ Arrhythmia Electrophysiol 2019;12(8):1–12.
10. Hayashi T, Santangeli P, Pathak RK, et al. Outcomes of catheter ablation of idiopathic outflow tract ventricular arrhythmias with an R wave pattern break in lead V2: a distinct clinical entity. J Cardiovasc Electrophysiol 2017;28(5):504–14.
11. Futyma P, Santangeli P, Pürerfellner H, et al. Anatomic approach with bipolar ablation between the left pulmonic cusp and left ventricular outflow tract for left ventricular summit arrhythmias. Heart Rhythm 2020;17(9):1519–27.
12. Santangeli P, Marchlinski FE, Zado ES, et al. Percutaneous epicardial ablation of ventricular arrhythmias arising from the left ventricular summit. Circ Arrhythmia Electrophysiol 2015;8(2):337–43.
13. Yamada T, Doppalapudi H, Maddox WR, et al. Prevalence and electrocardiographic and electrophysiological characteristics of idiopathic ventricular arrhythmias originating from intramural foci in the left ventricular outflow tract. Circ Arrhythmia Electrophysiol 2016;9(9):1–10.
14. Chung FP, Lin CY, Shirai Y, et al. Outcomes of catheter ablation of ventricular arrhythmia originating from the left ventricular summit: a multicenter study. Heart Rhythm 2020;17(7):1077–83. https://doi.org/10.1016/j.hrthm.2020.02.027. Available at:.

15. Berruezo A, Mont L, Nava S, et al. Electrocardio-graphic recognition of the epicardial origin of ventricular tachycardias. Circulation 2004;109(15):1842–7.
16. Vallès E, Bazan V, Marchlinski FE. ECG criteria to identify epicardial ventricular tachycardia in nonischemic cardiomyopathy. Circ Arrhythmia Electrophysiol 2010;3(1):63–71.
17. Yamada T, Murakami Y, Yoshida N, et al. Preferential conduction across the ventricular outflow septum in ventricular arrhythmias originating from the aortic sinus cusp. J Am Coll Cardiol 2007;50(9):884–91.

Predictors of Successful Endocardial Ablation of Epicardial Left Ventricular Summit Arrhythmias

Takumi Yamada, MD, PhD

KEYWORDS

- Anatomical approach • Endocardial • Left ventricular summit • Left ventricular outflow tract
- Radiofrequency catheter ablation • Ventricular arrhythmia

KEY POINTS

- Endocardial catheter ablation of ventricular arrhythmias (VAs) originating from the left ventricular summit (LVS) by an anatomic approach can be an alternative option, but it may not be so successful.
- A right bundle branch block pattern with a right inferior axis QRS morphology might be an electro-cardiographic predictor of a successful endocardial catheter ablation of LVS VAs.
- An endocardial catheter ablation of LVS VAs by an anatomic approach is successful most commonly in the left ventricular outflow tract followed by the aortic cusps and rarely in the right ventricular outflow tract.
- There are no electrophysiological predictors of a successful endocardial catheter ablation of LVS VAs.
- An anatomic distance between the earliest ventricular activation site in the coronary venous system and endocardial ablation site (<13 mm) could be a predictor of a successful endocardial catheter ablation of LVS VAs.

INTRODUCTION

Advances in electrophysiology and the technologies of catheter ablation, combined with a better understanding of the cardiac anatomy, have improved the outcome of catheter ablation of idiopathic ventricular arrhythmias (VAs).[1–11] Catheter ablation of idiopathic VAs is usually highly successful. However, when idiopathic VAs originate from the left ventricular summit (LVS), mapping and catheter ablation of those epicardial VAs remains challenging because of the anatomic barriers such as the close proximity to the coronary arteries and thick epicardial fat pads.[5,8,9,12–14] When it is not safe to deliver radiofrequency (RF)

energy directly to those VA foci or those VA foci cannot be reached because of anatomic barriers, an alternative approach from the endocardial side may be considered (anatomic approach).[8,9,15,16] In this approach, RF catheter ablation at an endocardial site remote from the LVS VA origins is expected to create an RF lesion large enough to reach those VA origins (**Fig. 1**). Anatomically, the endocardial structures adjacent to the LVS include the left coronary cusp (LCC), junction between the left and right coronary cusps (L-RCCs), left ventricular outflow tract (LVOT) including the aorto-mitral continuity (AMC), and right ventricular outflow tract (RVOT) (**Fig. 2**). Endocardial catheter ablation of LVS VAs by the

Cardiovascular Division, University of Minnesota, 420 Delaware Street Southeast, MMC 508, Minneapolis, MN 55455, USA
E-mail address: takumi-y@fb4.so-net.ne.jp

Card Electrophysiol Clin 15 (2023) 15–24
https://doi.org/10.1016/j.ccep.2022.04.005

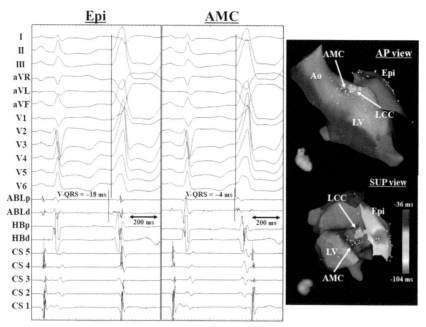

Fig. 1. Cardiac tracings exhibiting the local ventricular activation recorded from the epicardial surface (Epi) and aorto-mitral continuity (AMC) during a premature ventricular contraction (PVC) (left and middle panels) and electroanatomical maps exhibiting the successful ablation site (right panels). Note that the earliest ventricular activation during the PVC was recorded on the epicardial surface at the LVS. The yellow and red tags indicate the ablation sites within the left coronary cusp and successful ablation site at the AMC, respectively. ABL, ablation catheter; Ao, aorta; AP, anteroposterior; CS 1 to 5, the first (most distal) to fifth (most proximal) electrode pairs of the coronary sinus catheter; LV, left ventricle; SUP, superior; V-QRS, the local ventricular activation time relative to the QRS onset; X d, p, the distal and proximal electrode pairs of the relevant catheter. (*From* Yamada T, Doppalapudi H, Litovsky SH, McElderry HT, Kay GN. Challenging Radiofrequency Catheter Ablation of Idiopathic Ventricular Arrhythmias Originating From the Left Ventricular Summit Near the Left Main Coronary Artery. *Circ Arrhythm Electrophysiol.* 2016;9:e004202; with permission.)

anatomic approach can be successful at any of these locations, but the most successful location of this ablation should be determined based on the mapping results and anatomic consideration. In this article, predictors of a successful endocardial catheter ablation of epicardial LVS VAs are discussed.

ANATOMIC BACKGROUND

The LVS was defined based on fluoroscopy and coronary angiography as the region on the epicardial surface of the left ventricle (LV) near the bifurcation of the left main coronary artery that is bounded by an arc from the left anterior descending coronary artery superior to the first septal perforating branch anterior to the left circumflex coronary artery laterally.[5] Thus, the LVS is fan-shaped with the distance from the bifurcation of the left coronary arteries to the first septal perforator being its radius. The main trunk of the great cardiac vein (GCV) bisects the LVS into an upper portion that is not accessible to epicardial catheter

ablation due to the close proximity to the proximal left coronary arteries and a thick overlying epicardial fat and a lower portion that may be accessible to epicardial catheter ablation. The upper and lower portions of the LVS have been defined as the *inaccessible* and *accessible areas*, respectively, in a previous study.[5] The GCV usually runs through the LVS away from the bifurcation of the left main coronary artery but sometimes through the LVS near that.[17]

When LVS VAs originate from the *inaccessible area*, epicardial catheter ablation of those VAs is challenging and less likely to be successful whereas that of LVS VAs originating from the *accessible area* is very successful. On the other hand, endocardial catheter ablation by an anatomic approach may be more successful for LVS VAs originating from the *inaccessible area* than those from the *accessible area* for a couple of anatomic reasons. First, the LV muscle wall thickness tapers toward the LV base (see **Fig. 2**).[9] The thinner the LV muscle wall is, the more successful the endocardial RF catheter

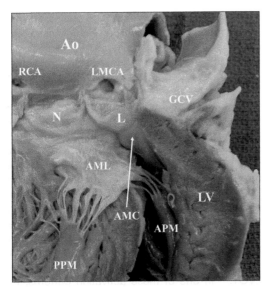

Fig. 2. An autopsy heart exhibiting the LVOT. AML, anterior mitral leaflet; APM, anterolateral papillary muscle; LCC, left coronary cusp; LMCA, left main coronary artery; N, noncoronary cusp; RCA, right coronary artery; PPM, posteromedial papillary muscle. The other abbreviations are as in the previous figure. (*From* Yamada T, Yoshida N, Doppalapudi H, Litovsky SH, McElderry HT, Kay GN. Efficacy of an Anatomical Approach in Radiofrequency Catheter Ablation of Idiopathic Ventricular Arrhythmias Originating From the Left Ventricular Outflow Tract. Circ Arrhythm Electrophysiol. 2017;10:e004959; with permission.)

ablation by an anatomic approach should be because there should be a better chance for that to create a transmural RF lesion reaching epicardial VA origins. Second, the *inaccessible area* can be approached from multiple endocardial sites including the LCC, L-RCC, and LVOT, whereas the *accessible area* can be approached only from the LVOT (see **Fig. 2**). An RF lesion from the LCC and L-RCC could reach epicardial LVS VA origins transversely, whereas that from the LVOT could do so vertically and transmurally.

ELECTROCARDIOGRAPHIC PREDICTORS

LVS VAs with a focal mechanism may exhibit characteristic electrocardiograms. Electrocardiographic characteristics may be helpful for predicting specific sites of those VA origins for which endocardial catheter ablation by an anatomic approach is more successful. Previous studies have suggested several electrocardiographic predictors of a successful endocardial catheter ablation of epicardial LVS arrhythmias. According to Yamada and colleagues'[9] study, a right

bundle branch block pattern with a right inferior axis QRS morphology was most prevalent in the successful group, whereas a left bundle branch block pattern with a right inferior axis QRS morphology was most prevalent in the unsuccessful group. A precordial transition of equal to or earlier than lead V1 was most prevalent in the successful group, whereas that between leads V2 and V3 was most prevalent in the unsuccessful group. Shirai and colleagues[16] also reported that a right bundle branch block pattern QRS morphology was significantly more prevalent in the successful group than the unsuccessful group. These electrocardiographic findings suggested that endocardial catheter ablation by an anatomic approach might have been more successful in VAs originating from the lateral portion of the LVS than the septal portion. These results could be well explained by the anatomic background. The LV muscle wall tapers toward the LV base attaching to the aorta and mitral annulus (see **Fig. 2**). The lateral side of the LVS faces the aorta and mitral annulus. Therefore, there would be a better chance for an RF lesion from the endocardial side to extend transmurally to reach the epicardial LVS VA origins in the lateral LVS than in the septal LVS. Yamada and colleagues[9] also reported that the maximal deflection index (MDI)[18] was significantly greater in the unsuccessful group than in the successful group. It has been reported that an MDI of greater than 0.55 might suggest epicardial VA origins.[18] Therefore, a greater MDI might suggest a larger distance from the endocardial surface to epicardial VA origins, which results in an unsuccessful endocardial catheter ablation of LVS VAs.

MAPPING OF LEFT VENTRICULAR SUMMIT VENTRICULAR ARRHYTHMIAS
Activation Mapping

The target sites of endocardial catheter ablation of LVS VAs by the anatomic approach should be determined by the localization of those VA origins. Activation mapping seeking the earliest bipolar activity and/or a local unipolar QS pattern during VAs is most reliable for identifying a site of a focal VA origin.[19] However, the anatomic barrier around the LVS might render activation mapping of LVS VAs less reliable. Mapping in adjacent structures such as the LCC, L-RCC, and LVOT including the AMC, RVOT, and coronary venous system (CVS) including the GCV is routinely performed to identify the sites of LVS VA origins. Because anatomically, the GCV runs through the LVS, the earliest ventricular activation is most commonly recorded within the GCV.[5,8,9,13,15–17] Recently, mapping of the small branches of the GCV such as the communicating branch with a multielectrode microcatheter has proven helpful for comprehensive mapping of LVS VAs.[20] However, this mapping does not cover the entire LVS area. Epicardial mapping through a trans-pericardial approach cannot achieve high-resolution mapping in this region. Therefore, the earliest ventricular activation recorded by this activation mapping does not always indicate a site of an LVS VA origin. There are no definite criteria of the local ventricular activation time that indicates a site of an LVS VA origin, but if the local ventricular activation does not precede the QRS onset by greater than 20 milliseconds, the LVS VA origins are unlikely to be located at that recording site. If LVS VAs are transiently suppressed by an RF ablation at the earliest ventricular activation site, those VA origins are likely to be located around that site.

Ventricular activation recorded from the endocardial structures adjacent to the LVS is often equal to or later than the QRS onset and is later than that recorded from the CVS during LVS VAs (**Figs. 3** and **4**). Therefore, activation mapping within those endocardial structures could not exactly identify the sites of LVS VA origins. However, activation patterns recorded within those endocardial structures might suggest a presumed site of an LVS VA origin.[17] When a centrifugal activation pattern is recorded in the LVOT during LVS VAs, the sites of those VA origins are suggested to be located at the epicardial site opposite the earliest endocardial ventricular activation site in the LVOT (see **Figs. 3** and **4**). That is because in such a setting, the ventricular activation from the LVS VA origins likely conducts transmurally through a relatively thin LV wall to the endocardial LVOT (**Fig. 5**). When LVS VAs present with an endocardial ventricular activation pattern from the LV base (AMC) toward the LV apex, a presumed site of the LVS VA origin should be speculated by considering two types of eccentric activation patterns from those origins to the LVOT.[17] In one of those activation patterns, the ventricular activation from the VA origin in the basal LVS does not spread radially with the transmural conduction from the VA origin to the AMC being slower than the epicardial conduction from the basal LVS VA origin to the GCV in the apical

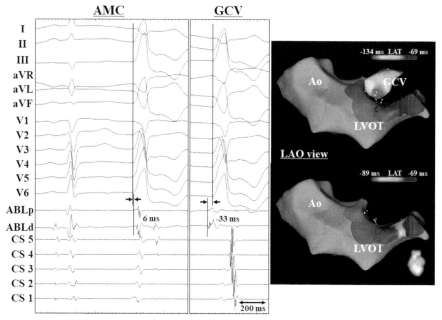

Fig. 3. Cardiac tracings exhibiting the local ventricular activations recorded in the AMC (left panel) and GCV (middle panel) and activation maps with and without the GCV recorded during the PVCs (right upper and lower panels, respectively). The catheter ablation was successful in the apical LVOT just below the GCV where the earliest ventricular activation was recorded. Note that the earliest endocardial ventricular activation was recorded at the successful ablation site in the apical LVOT, from where the activation propagated toward the AMC. The red tag indicates the successful ablation site. LAO, left anterior oblique; LAT, local activation time. The other abbreviations are as in the previous figures. (*From* Yamada T, Kumar V, Yoshida N, Doppalapudi H. Eccentric activation patterns in the left ventricular outflow tract during idiopathic ventricular arrhythmias originating from the left ventricular summit: A pitfall for predicting the sites of ventricular arrhythmia origins. Circ Arrhythm Electrophysiol. 2019;12:e007419; with permission.)

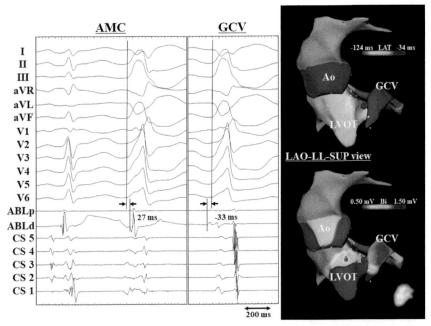

Fig. 4. Cardiac tracings exhibiting the local ventricular activations recorded in the AMC (left panel) and GCV (middle panel) and activation and voltage maps recorded during the PVCs (right panels). The catheter ablation was successful in the GCV where the earliest ventricular activation was recorded. Note that the earliest endocardial ventricular activation was recorded in the apical LVOT just below the GCV, from where the activation propagated toward the AMC. The red tag indicates the successful ablation site. Bi, bipolar electrogram amplitude; LL, left lateral. The other abbreviations are as in the previous figures. (*From* Yamada T, Kumar V, Yoshida N, Doppalapudi H. Eccentric activation patterns in the left ventricular outflow tract during idiopathic ventricular arrhythmias originating from the left ventricular summit: A pitfall for predicting the sites of ventricular arrhythmia origins. Circ Arrhythm Electrophysiol. 2019;12:e007419; with permission.)

LVS (see **Fig. 5**; **Fig. 6**). In the other activation pattern, the ventricular activation from VA origins in the apical LVS propagates epicardially toward the LV base, whereas the endocardial activation pattern during those VAs is from the AMC to the apical LVOT (see **Fig. 5**; **Fig. 7**). It should be noted that the first activation pattern can occur more often than the second one. When a relatively early ventricular activation is recorded from multiple separated structures around the LVS, such LVS VA origins might be located in the middle between those locations (**Fig. 8**).

Pace Mapping

Pace mapping may be helpful, when VAs are infrequent during mapping and ablation and roughly localize the site of the VA origin.[19] Pace mapping may be less helpful for LVS VAs because pacing within the CVS may not exactly reproduce the QRS morphology of the VAs or obtain myocardial capture despite the use of high pacing current. If pace maps from the earliest ventricular activation site within the CVS highly match the LVS VAs, those VA origins are likely to be located at that site. However, it should be noted that highly matched pace maps do not always indicate sites of LVS VA origins when there is a preferential conduction from the VA origin to breakout sites (see **Fig. 6**).[17] Pace mapping from the endocardial sites is unlikely to be helpful for determining a target site of an endocardial catheter ablation of LVS VAs by the anatomic approach.

PREDICTORS OF SUCCESSFUL ENDOCARDIAL ABLATION OF EPICARDIAL LEFT VENTRICULAR SUMMIT ARRHYTHMIAS

It might be challenging to detect the success rate of the endocardial catheter ablation of LVS VAs alone by an anatomic approach because the current mapping technologies cannot differentiate LVS VA origins from intramural LVOT VA origins accurately when the endocardial catheter ablation is successful.[9,16] Shirai and colleagues and Yamada and colleagues reported that the endocardial catheter ablation by an anatomic approach was successful in 49% and 55% of the overall VAs originating from the ventricular outflow tract with the earliest ventricular

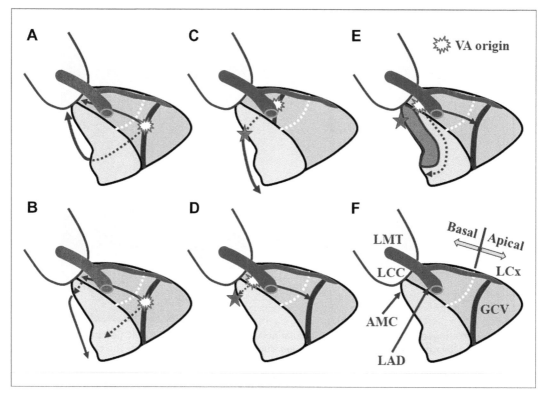

Fig. 5. Diagrams exhibiting the LV summit with the adjacent anatomic structures and activation patterns in the LVOT. (*A*) A normal activation pattern with a VA origin in the apical LV summit. (*B*) An eccentric activation pattern with a VA origin in the apical LV summit. (*C*) A normal activation pattern with a VA origin in the basal LV summit. Note that the GCV runs through the basal LV summit. (*D*) An eccentric activation pattern with a VA origin in the basal LV summit. (*E*) An eccentric activation pattern with a VA origin in the basal LV summit and endocardial scar (brown area). (*F*) The anatomic structures are labeled. The stars indicate the successful ablation sites on the endocardial side. The black solid and dotted arrows in the diagrams of A through E indicate the activation propagating along the endocardial or epicardial surface and through the intramural region, respectively. LAD, left anterior descending coronary artery; LCx, left circumflex coronary artery; LMT, left main trunk. The other abbreviations are as in the previous figures. (*From* Yamada T, Kumar V, Yoshida N, Doppalapudi H. Eccentric activation patterns in the left ventricular outflow tract during idiopathic ventricular arrhythmias originating from the left ventricular summit: A pitfall for predicting the sites of ventricular arrhythmia origins. Circ Arrhythm Electrophysiol. 2019;12:e007419; with permission.)

activation within the CVS, respectively.[9,16] Yamada and colleagues[9] reported that the endocardial catheter ablation by an anatomic approach was successful in 77% and 25% of intramural LVOT VAs and LVS VAs, respectively, based on their own criteria for differentiating those VAs. Therefore, the endocardial catheter ablation of LVS VAs by an anatomic approach may not be so successful.

The endocardial catheter ablation of LVS VAs by an anatomic approach is successful most commonly in the LVOT followed by the aortic cusps and rarely in the RVOT.[9,16] Endocardial catheter ablation from multiple sites is sometimes required for a successful ablation of LVS VAs.[16] It should depend on multiple factors including the

distribution of the LVS VA origins, ventricular muscle wall thickness, accuracy of the localization of those VA origins, and so forth, where this endocardial catheter ablation is successful. However, when the LVOT is suggested to be the best target of the endocardial catheter ablation of LVS VAs, there might be a better chance for a successful ablation as compared with the other locations.

An accurate localization of LVS VA origins and the formation of an RF lesion that can reach those VA origins can make endocardial catheter ablation of LVS VAs by the anatomic approach successful. As mentioned above, an accurate localization of the LVS VA origins is often challenging, but it should be the first key for a

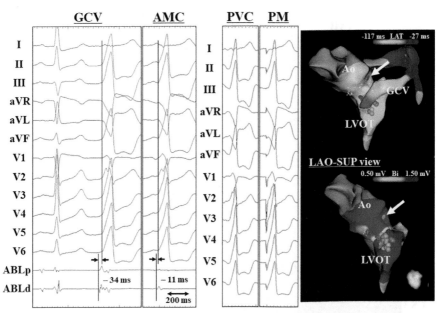

Fig. 6. Cardiac tracings exhibiting the local ventricular activations recorded in the GCV and AMC (left panels) and a PVC and pace map (PM) (middle panels), and the activation and voltage maps recorded during the PVCs (right panels). The catheter ablation was unsuccessful in the apical LVOT just below the GCV where the earliest ventricular activation was recorded. The catheter ablation was successful in the AMC (*arrows*) where the earliest endocardial ventricular activation was recorded. The pink and red tags indicate the ablation sites. Note that an excellent PM was demonstrated in the GCV away from the successful ablation site. The abbreviations are as in the previous figures. (*From* Yamada T, Kumar V, Yoshida N, Doppalapudi H. Eccentric activation patterns in the left ventricular outflow tract during idiopathic ventricular arrhythmias originating from the left ventricular summit: A pitfall for predicting the sites of ventricular arrhythmia origins. Circ Arrhythm Electrophysiol. 2019;12:e007419; with permission.)

successful endocardial catheter ablation of LVS VAs. Creation of a deep and most likely transmural RF lesion is required for a successful endocardial catheter ablation of LVS VAs. To create such an RF lesion, a long duration of a high RF energy delivery is usually applied. Use of half-normal saline as an irrigant[21] may enhance such an irrigated RF lesion with a better outcome of endocardial catheter ablation of LVS VAs, but there has been no evidence to prove that.

Because the size of the RF lesion is limited, an identification of an optimal ablation target site should be the second key for a successful endocardial catheter ablation of LVS VAs. Shirai and colleagues[16] investigated whether any electrophysiological and anatomic relationships between the earliest ventricular activation site in the CVS and endocardial ablation site could predict a successful endocardial catheter ablation of LVS VAs and revealed that only an anatomic distance between those two sites might be its predictor. In their study, there was some degree of overlap in the anatomic distance between the successful and unsuccessful groups, but a cut-off distance of greater than 12.8 mm strongly

predicted failure of an endocardial catheter ablation by the anatomic approach. Another study from the same group reported that a cut-off of less than 13.5 mm for the anatomic distance between the earliest ventricular activation site in the CVS and targeted endocardial site had a reasonable sensitivity and specificity to predict a successful ablation.[15] It should be noted that such an anatomic distance does not indicate the real distance between the VA origins and endocardial ablation site for several reasons. First, the site of the earliest ventricular activation is not always the site of the LVS VA origin. Therefore, when endocardial catheter ablation of LVS VAs is unsuccessful at a short distance from the earliest ventricular activation site in the CVS, those VA origins are likely to be located away from the earliest ventricular activation site. Second, the CVS usually runs through the epicardial fat pad in the LVS, and there should be a fat layer intervening between the CVS and epicardial surface (see **Fig. 2**). Therefore, if there is a thick fat layer between the CVS and epicardial VA origins, endocardial catheter ablation of LVS VAs may be successful at a long distance

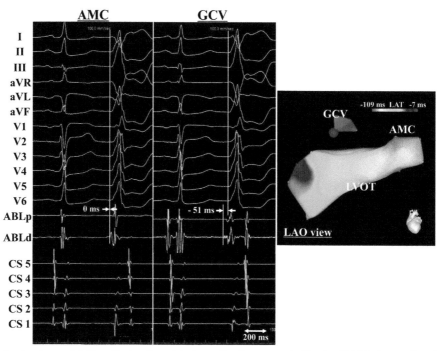

Fig. 7. Cardiac tracings exhibiting the local ventricular activations recorded in the AMC (left panel) and GCV (middle panel), and the activation map recorded during the PVCs (right panel). The catheter ablation was successful in the GCV where the earliest ventricular activation was recorded. Note that the endocardial ventricular activation pattern was from the AMC to the apical LVOT. The red tag indicates the successful ablation site. The abbreviations are as in the previous figures. (*From* Yamada T, Kumar V, Yoshida N, Doppalapudi H. Eccentric activation patterns in the left ventricular outflow tract during idiopathic ventricular arrhythmias originating from the left ventricular summit: A pitfall for predicting the sites of ventricular arrhythmia origins. Circ Arrhythm Electrophysiol. 2019;12:e007419; with permission.)

from the earliest ventricular activation site in the CVS.

The anatomic distance between the LVS VA origins and endocardial ablation site cannot be determined accurately because of the intervening epicardial fat layer. The difference in the activation time between the earliest ventricular activation site in the CVS and endocardial ablation site might be considered more helpful for predicting a successful endocardial catheter ablation of LVS VAs because that should reflect the time for the ventricular activation to travel between those two sites and might be better correlated to the real distance between the LVS VA origins and endocardial ablation site than the anatomic distance mentioned above. However, Shirai and colleagues[16] reported that the difference in the activation time did not significantly differ between the successful and unsuccessful groups. This finding may be explained not only by an inaccurate localization of the LVS VA origins but also by varied transmural conduction properties including preferential conduction.

SUMMARY

When it is not safe to deliver RF energy directly to LVS VA foci or those VA foci cannot be reached because of anatomic barriers, endocardial catheter ablation from remote structures adjacent to the LVS may be considered as an alternative option (anatomic approach). However, such endocardial catheter ablation of LVS VAs by an anatomic approach may not be so successful. The endocardial catheter ablation of LVS VAs by an anatomic approach is successful most commonly in the LVOT followed by the aortic cusps and rarely in the RVOT. A right bundle branch block pattern with a right inferior axis QRS morphology might be an electrocardiographic predictor of a successful endocardial catheter ablation of LVS VAs. There are no electrophysiological predictors of a successful endocardial catheter ablation of LVS VAs. The anatomic distance between the earliest ventricular activation site in the CVS and endocardial ablation site (<13 mm) could be a predictor of a successful endocardial catheter ablation of LVS VAs.

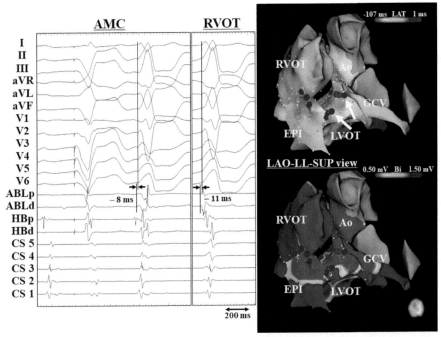

Fig. 8. Cardiac tracings exhibiting the local ventricular activations recorded in the AMC (left panel) and RVOT (middle panel), and the activation and voltage maps recorded during the PVCs (right panels). The earliest ventricular activation (around −10 msec relative to the QRS onset) was recorded at multiple sites such as the apical LVOT, GCV, RVOT, and left ventricular epicardial surface (EPI), but the catheter ablation was successful at the junction between the left and right coronary cusps. Note that an endocardial low-voltage area extended further to the apical LVOT than the other cases. The red and blue tags indicate the successful and unsuccessful ablation sites, respectively. The other abbreviations are as in the previous figures. (*From* Yamada T, Kumar V, Yoshida N, Doppalapudi H. Eccentric activation patterns in the left ventricular outflow tract during idiopathic ventricular arrhythmias originating from the left ventricular summit: A pitfall for predicting the sites of ventricular arrhythmia origins. Circ Arrhythm Electrophysiol. 2019;12:e007419; with permission.)

CLINICS CARE POINTS

1. Endocardial catheter ablation of left ventricular summit (LVS) ventricular arrhythmias (VAs) by an anatomic approach can be an alternative option, but it may not be so successful.

2. A right bundle branch block pattern with a right inferior axis QRS morphology might be an electrocardiographic predictor of a successful endocardial catheter ablation of LVS VAs.

3. An accurate localization of LVS VA origins is often challenging, but it should be the first key for a successful endocardial catheter ablation of LVS VAs.

4. Activation mapping seeking the earliest ventricular activation is a gold standard to localize LVS VA origins, but the endocardial activation pattern might be helpful for predicting sites of those VAs.

5. The identification of an optimal ablation target site should be the second key for a successful endocardial catheter ablation of LVS VAs because the size of radiofrequency lesion is limited.

6. An endocardial catheter ablation of LVS VAs by an anatomic approach is successful most commonly in the left ventricular outflow tract followed by the aortic cusps and rarely in the right ventricular outflow tract.

7. There are no electrophysiological predictors of a successful endocardial catheter ablation of LVS VAs.

8. An anatomic distance between the earliest ventricular activation site in the coronary venous system and endocardial ablation site of less than 13 mm could be a predictor of a successful endocardial catheter ablation of LVS VAs.

DISCLOSURE

None.

REFERENCES

1. Stevenson WG, Soejima K. Catheter ablation for ventricular tachycardia. Circulation 2007;115: 2750–60.
2. Yamada T, Yoshida N, Murakami Y, et al. Electrocardiographic characteristics of ventricular arrhythmias originating from the junction of the left and right coronary sinuses of Valsalva in the aorta: the activation pattern as a rationale for the electrocardiographic characteristics. Heart Rhythm 2008;5:184–92.
3. Yamada T, McElderry HT, Doppalapudi H, et al. Idiopathic ventricular arrhythmias originating from the aortic root: prevalence, electrocardiographic and electrophysiological characteristics, and results of the radiofrequency catheter ablation. J Am Coll Cardiol 2008;52:139–47.
4. Yamada T, Litovsky SH, Kay GN. The left ventricular ostium: an anatomic concept relevant to idiopathic ventricular arrhythmias. Circ Arrhythmia Electrophysiol 2008;1:396–404.
5. Yamada T, McElderry HT, Doppalapudi H, et al. Idiopathic ventricular arrhythmias originating from the left ventricular summit: anatomic concepts relevant to ablation. Circ Arrhythm Electrophysiol 2010;3: 616–23.
6. Yamada T, Maddox WR, McElderry HT, et al. Radiofrequency catheter ablation of idiopathic ventricular arrhythmias originating from intramural foci in the left ventricular outflow tract; efficacy of sequential vs. simultaneous unipolar catheter ablation. Circ Arrhythm Electrophysiol 2015;8:344–52.
7. Yamada T, Doppalapudi H, Maddox WR, et al. Prevalence and electrocardiographic and electrophysiological characteristics of idiopathic ventricular arrhythmias originating from intramural foci in the left ventricular outflow tract. Circ Arrhythm Electrophysiol 2016;9:e004079.
8. Yamada T, Doppalapudi H, Litovsky SH, et al. Challenging radiofrequency catheter ablation of idiopathic ventricular arrhythmias originating from the left ventricular summit near the left main coronary artery. Circ Arrhythm Electrophysiol 2016;9:e004202.
9. Yamada T, Yoshida N, Doppalapudi H, et al. Efficacy of an anatomical approach in radiofrequency catheter ablation of idiopathic ventricular arrhythmias originating from the left ventricular outflow tract. Circ Arrhythm Electrophysiol 2017;10:e004959.
10. Yamada T, Yoshida N, Itoh T, et al. Idiopathic ventricular arrhythmias originating from the parietal band: electrocardiographic and electrophysiological
characteristics and outcome of catheter ablation. Circ Arrhythm Electrophysiol 2017;10:e005099.
11. Yamada T, Yoshida N, Litovsky SH, et al. Idiopathic ventricular arrhythmias originating from the infundibular muscles: prevalence, electrocardiographic and electrophysiological characteristics, and outcome of catheter ablation. Circ Arrhythm Electrophysiol 2018;11:e005749.
12. Yamada T. Transthoracic epicardial catheter ablation: indications, techniques, and complications. Circ J 2013;77:1672–80.
13. Santangeli P, Marchlinski FE, Zado ES, et al. Percutaneous epicardial ablation of ventricular arrhythmias arising from the left ventricular summit: outcomes and electrocardiogram correlates of success. Circ Arrhythm Electrophysiol 2015;8:337–43.
14. Carrigan TP, Patel S, Yokokawa M, et al. Anatomic relationships between the coronary venous system, surrounding structures, and the site of origin of epicardial ventricular arrhythmias. J Cardiovasc Electrophysiol 2014;25:1336–42.
15. Jauregui Abularach ME, Campos B, Park KM, et al. Ablation of ventricular arrhythmias arising near the anterior epicardial veins from the left sinus of Valsalva region: ECG features, anatomic distance, and outcome. Heart Rhythm 2012;9:865–73.
16. Shirai Y, Santangeli P, Liang JJ, et al. Anatomical proximity dictates successful ablation from adjacent sites for outflow tract ventricular arrhythmias linked to the coronary venous system. Europace 2019;21:484–91.
17. Yamada T, Kumar V, Yoshida N, et al. Eccentric activation patterns in the left ventricular outflow tract during idiopathic ventricular arrhythmias originating from the left ventricular summit: a pitfall for predicting the sites of ventricular arrhythmia origins. Circ Arrhythm Electrophysiol 2019;12:e007419.
18. Daniels DV, Lu YY, Morton JB, et al. Idiopathic epicardial left ventricular tachycardia originating remote from the sinus of Valsalva: electrophysiological characteristics, catheter ablation, and identification from the 12-lead electrocardiogram. Circulation 2006;113:1659–66.
19. Yamada T, Kay GN. Optimal ablation strategies for different types of ventricular tachycardias. Nat Rev Cardiol 2012;9:512–25.
20. Komatsu Y, Nogami A, Shinoda Y, et al. Idiopathic ventricular arrhythmias originating from the vicinity of the communicating vein of cardiac venous systems at the left ventricular summit. Circ Arrhythm Electrophysiol 2018;11:e005386.
21. Nguyen DT, Gerstenfeld EP, Tzou WS, et al. Radiofrequency ablation using an open irrigated electrode cooled with half-normal saline. JACC Clin Electrophysiol 2017;3:1103–10.

Percutaneous Epicardial Ablation of Ventricular Arrhythmias Arising from the Left Ventricular Summit

Yasuhiro Shirai, MD, PhD

KEYWORDS

- Percutaneous epicardial mapping and ablation • Left ventricular summit
- Outflow tract ventricular arrhythmia • Electrocardiogram

KEY POINTS

- Direct epicardial ablation of outflow tract ventricular arrhythmias arising from the left ventricular summit is successful only in a minority of patients.
- Direct epicardial ablation can be successful only when the site of origin is localized at the base of the left ventricular summit (accessible area) apart from the coronary vessels and thick fat layer.
- Electrocardiographic characteristics are useful for predicting the site of origin within the left ventricular summit, and needs to be evaluated before performing epicardial mapping after failed alternative ablation strategy.

BACKGROUND

The left ventricular summit (LVS) is the highest point of the left ventricular epicardium, and ventricular arrhythmias (VA) originating from this area accounts for 10% to 15% of idiopathic outflow tract VA (OTVA).[1] Because the target of ablation should be at epicardial surface when OTVA arise from the LVS, direct epicardial mapping and ablation by performing pericardiocentesis might be effective. However, epicardial ablation involves higher risk compared with endocardial ablation and the efficacy of direct epicardial ablation is limited because of the epicardial vessels that run the LVS area and the epicardial fat.

MAPPING FEATURES AND ABLATION OUTCOME

Santangeli and colleagues[2] recently reported a series of 23 consecutive patients who underwent percutaneous epicardial mapping of VA arising from the LVS. In their series, percutaneous epicardial mapping was performed after failed ablation from multiple adjacent locations including the left ventricular/right ventricular endocardium, the aortic sinus of Valsalva, and within the coronary venous system (CVS). Furthermore, epicardial activation or pace mapping confirmed origin of the VA from the LVS in all patients. In this study, epicardial ablation was attempted only in 14 (61%) out of 23 patients; in the remaining nine (39%) cases, radiofrequency energy application was aborted because of close proximity to either left anterior descending (LAD) or circumflex (LCX) coronary artery. Furthermore, the targeted VA was acutely suppressed in only 5 (22%) out of 14 patients in whom direct epicardial ablation was performed.

In another case series by Yamada and his colleagues,[1] epicardial mapping and ablation was attempted in 9 out of 27 patients with LVS VA, which was determined by successful catheter ablation or presumed by electrophysiologic study. In this study, percutaneous epicardial mapping was performed after unsuccessful ablation from adjacent locations including the CVS in four out

Department of Cardiology, Disaster Medical Center, 3256 Midoricho Tachikawa, Tokyo, Japan
E-mail address: whity_yasuo@yahoo.co.jp

Card Electrophysiol Clin 15 (2023) 25–30
https://doi.org/10.1016/j.ccep.2022.07.002
1877-9182/23/© 2022 Elsevier Inc. All rights reserved.

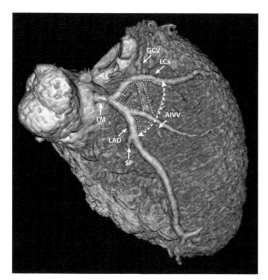

Fig. 1. Computed tomographic image of the left ventricular summit. The left ventricular summit (defined as the triangular portion of the epicardial left ventricular outflow tract with the apex at the bifurcation between the LAD and LCX and the base formed by an arc connecting the first septal perforator with the LCX) is bisected by the GCV into two regions: one closer to the apex of the triangle (inaccessible area), and one at the base of the triangle (accessible area). The *blue dotted area* indicates inaccessible area and the *yellow dotted area* indicates accessible area within the left ventricular summit. AIVV, anterior interventricular vein; GCV, great cardiac vein; LM, left main coronary artery; SP, septal perforator. (*From* Santangeli P, Marchlinski FE, Zado ES, et al. Percutaneous epicardial ablation of ventricular arrhythmias arising from the left ventricular summit: outcomes and electrocardiogram correlates of success. Circ Arrhythm Electrophysiol;8:337–343; with permission.)

of nine patients. In the remaining five patients, activation map (including within the CVS) did not reveal any early local ventricular activation and epicardial mapping was conducted. Of these nine patients, successful ablation was achieved on the epicardial surface in four (44%) patients and epicardial ablation was abandoned in the remaining five patients because of close proximity to the coronary artery or high impedance.

Of note, the VA were localized at the base of the LVS triangle (lateral and posterior aspect of the LVS) in all the successful cases in both studies. The LVS (defined as the triangular portion of the epicardial LVOT with the apex at the bifurcation between the LAD and the LCX and the base formed by an arc connecting the first septal perforator with the LCX) is bisected by the great cardiac vein into two regions: one closer to the apex of the triangle and one at the base of the triangle (**Fig. 1**).

Because the apex of the triangle is closer to major coronary arteries (**Fig. 2**) and is covered with a thick layer of epicardial fat, this region is defined as the inaccessible area where catheter ablation is unlikely to be successful. However, VA arising from the base of the LVS triangle (accessible area) is amenable to percutaneous epicardial ablation as long as the distance between the site of origin and the coronary vessel is convincingly safe.

ELECTROCARDIOGRAM CHARACTERISTICS

As shown in the previous studies, the efficacy of percutaneous epicardial ablation is limited especially when the site of origin is located in the inaccessible area of the LVS.[1,2] In this regard, preprocedural planning for ablation strategy is important to avoid unnecessary pericardiocentesis. Because the inaccessible area is located more anteromedial compared with the accessible area, which is located in the posterolateral portion of the LVS, electrocardiographic (ECG) characteristics are useful to predict the site of origin (and accordingly ablation outcome) within the LVS.

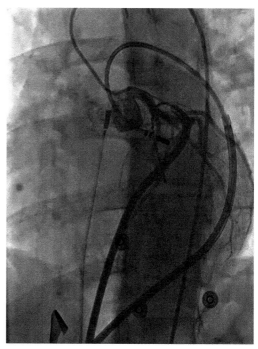

Fig. 2. Anatomic proximity between the apex of the left ventricular summit and major coronary arteries. Left anterior oblique view of the fluoroscopic image showing a multielectrode catheter inside the anterior interventricular vein and an ablation catheter over the earliest premature ventricular contraction (PVC) activation during left coronarography. (*Courtesy of* Luis C. Sáenz, MD, Bogota, Colombia.)

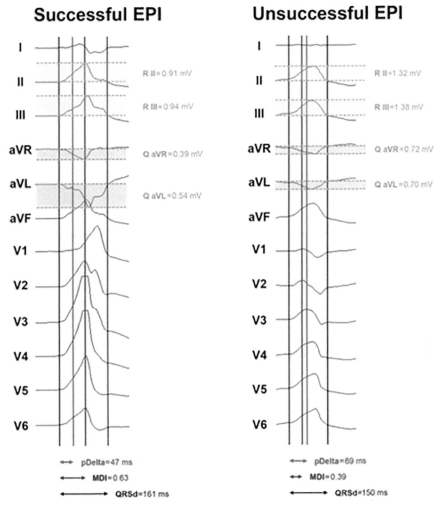

Successful EPI

I

II   R II = 0.91 mV

III   R III = 0.94 mV

aVR   Q aVR = 0.39 mV

aVL   Q aVL = 0.54 mV

aVF

V1

V2

V3

V4

V5

V6

⟷ pDelta = 47 ms
⟷ MDI = 0.63
⟷ QRSd = 161 ms

Unsuccessful EPI

I

II   R II = 1.32 mV

III   R III = 1.38 mV

aVR   Q aVR = 0.72 mV

aVL   Q aVL = 0.70 mV

aVF

V1

V2

V3

V4

V5

V6

⟷ pDelta = 69 ms
⟷ MDI = 0.39
⟷ QRSd = 150 ms

Fig. 3. Comparison of ECG measurements in a sample patient with successful epicardial ablation and in one with unsuccessful ablation. MDI, maximum deflection index; QRSd, QRS duration. (*From* Santangeli P, Marchlinski FE, Zado ES, et al. Percutaneous epicardial ablation of ventricular arrhythmias arising from the left ventricular summit: outcomes and electrocardiogram correlates of success. Circ Arrhythm Electrophysiol; 8:337–343; with permission.)

In the case series by Santangeli and colleagues,[2] comparison of ECG characteristics between patients with successful epicardial ablation and those with unsuccessful ablation (including patients in whom epicardial ablation was abandoned) was reported. According to their study, a right bundle branch block morphology of the VA was present in four (80%) out of five successful cases, whereas 9 (50%) out of 18 unsuccessful cases. In patients exhibiting left bundle branch block morphology, the Q-wave ratio in leads aVL/aVR was the only parameter that was significantly different between the successful and unsuccessful group. The Q-wave ratio in leads aVL/aVR was significantly greater in patients with successful epicardial ablation than that in the

unsuccessful group (2.63 ± 1.31 vs 1.39 ± 0.58, respectively; $P = 0.017$). Although not statistically significant, other ECG characteristics indicating lateral site of origin within the LVS area, such as a QS complex in lead I, absence of an initial q wave in lead V_1, and an R-wave to S-wave ratio in lead $V_1 > V_2$, were more frequently present in successful epicardial ablation group. Based on these findings, they suggested three ECG criteria to help identify patients who had successful epicardial ablation: (1) Q-wave ratio in leads aVL/aVR >1.85, (2) R/S-wave ratio in lead $V_1 > V_2$, and (3) lack of initial q wave in lead V_1 (**Fig. 3**). The presence of at least two of these three ECG criteria was associated with successful epicardial ablation with 100% sensitivity and 72% specificity

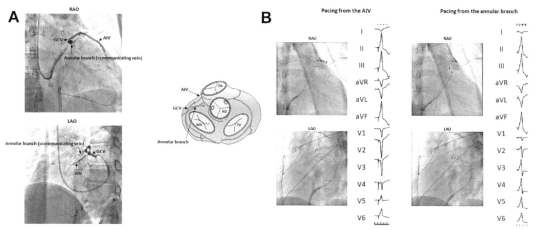

Fig. 4. Unique ECG patterns demonstrated by pace mapping within the left ventricular summit. (*A*) Coronary sinus venography shows the main trunk (the GCV and the AIV) and the annular branch (communicating branch) on the *left*. The *right* schema represents the anatomic relationship between the coronary venous system and the ventricular outflow tract. Although AIV runs the anterior interventricular sulcus along the LAD, the annular branch, also labeled as "communicating branch," arises before the GCV-AIV junction and runs toward the septum in the LAO projection and is completely foreshortened in the RAO projection by overlapping the GCV. (*B*) When paced from the electrodes within the AIV, which runs along the LAD, V_2 pattern break was reproduced, whereas abrupt V_3 transition was reproducible when pace map was performed at the electrodes within the annular branch (communicating branch), which runs septal and basal aspect of the LVS. The *red arrowheads* represent the paced electrodes within the AIV (*left*) and the annular branch (*right*). AIV, anterior interventricular vein; LAO, left anterior oblique; RAO, right anterior oblique.

in their study. As for the ECG characteristics, Yamada and colleagues[1] also reported that the Q-wave ratio in leads aVL/aVR and the R-wave ratio in leads III/II were significantly greater in the group of patients with VA from accessible area, which was consistent with the results by Santangeli and colleagues.[2]

Other ECG characteristics suggesting the LVS origin, which was reported recently, includes V_2 pattern break and abrupt V_3 transition.[3,4] Hayashi and colleagues[3] identified 12 (9%) cases with pattern break in lead V_2 out of 130 consecutive OTVA (with left bundle branch morphology) patients. The pattern break in V_2 was defined as net QRS amplitude in lead V_2 being less positive or having a smaller R wave than in lead V_1 and V_3. Because the location of lead V_2 electrodes often corresponds to the anterior interventricular sulcus, the site of origin of the VA was located near the LAD and ablation was abandoned in almost half of the patients with V_2 pattern break. Although ablation was acutely successful from adjacent sites including the anterior-septal right ventricular OT or the left coronary cusp in the remaining patients with V_2 pattern break, the recurrence rate during follow-up remained high. According to their data, VA elimination was achieved in 58% of patients with V_2 pattern break compared with 89% of the reference population. In their series, epicardial mapping via subxiphoid access was

performed in 3 out of 12 patients with V_2 pattern break and the earliest activation was recorded in 2 patients. For the two patients, ablation could not be performed on the epicardium because of anatomic proximity to the coronary artery and VA elimination was not achieved. Another unique ECG pattern, abrupt V_3 transition, was reported by Liao and his colleagues.[4] Of 78 consecutive OTVA patients, they identified 20 (26%) patients with abrupt V_3 transition, which was defined as R-wave amplitude in lead V_3 three-times greater than that in lead V_2 with a precordial transition at lead V_3. They hypothesized that the sudden transition at V_3 was caused by activation in a posterior direction away from lead V_1 and V_2, with inferior and leftward activation directed toward lead V_3, which is indicative of a site of origin from the septal margin of the LVS. In their series of 20 patients with abrupt V_3 transition, the earliest activation was recorded at the right-left aortic interleaflet triangle in 10, great cardiac vein/anterior interventricular vein in four, epicardium at the proximal LAD artery in two, intramural in three, and aortomitral continuity in one. The successful ablation site was right-left aortic interleaflet triangle, which corresponds to the septal margin of the LVS in 16 (80%). Of note, ablation by the robotic epicardial approach was required in two patients. Based on the results from these recent studies, V_2 pattern break and abrupt V_3 transition are suggestive of a site of origin from inaccessible area of the LVS. **Fig. 4** demonstrates these unique ECG patterns by pace mapping findings from the CVS. When paced from the electrodes within the anterior interventricular vein, which runs along the LAD, V_2 pattern break was reproduced, whereas, abrupt V_3 transition was reproducible when pace map was performed at the electrodes within the annular branch (communicating branch), which runs septal and basal aspect of the LVS. As shown in **Fig. 4**, although both ECG patterns are associated with septal aspect of the LVS where epicardial ablation is unlikely to be successful, anatomically adjacent site to the site of origin would be anterior-septal right ventricular OT for the VA with V_2 pattern break and the LVOT including the aortic sinus of Valsalva for the VA with abrupt V_3 transition.

DISCUSSION

The efficacy of direct epicardial mapping and ablation is limited as shown in the previous case series described here.[1,2] The multicenter study, which is the largest series of patients with OTVAs from the LVS, has recently been reported by Chung and colleagues.[5] In this multicenter study, overall acute success rate was 84% (199) of 238 patients with VA from the LVS. Among 199 patients with successful ablation, success site was on epicardium in 19 (9.5%) patients. As such, success rate turned out to be improved from 76% to 84% (+8%) by performing direct epicardial mapping and ablation in this study. However, it is important to recognize that epicardial ablation within the LVS is available only when the site of origin is apart from the coronary vessels and is not covered by epicardial fat. Although the indication for direct epicardial mapping via subxiphoid access is different between each previous study, radiofrequency energy application on the epicardium was available in approximately only half of the patients in whom direct epicardial mapping was performed. In this regard, it is important to consider whether the site of origin is located within the accessible area of the LVS by evaluating the ECG characteristics described previously to avoid ineffective epicardial approach. Epicardial approach might be considered after failed alternative ablation strategy only when the ECG morphology is favorable for successful epicardial ablation and the benefit outweighs the risk.

Alternative ablation strategies for the OTVA from the LVS includes radiofrequency ablation within the CVS,[6] anatomic approach targeting the adjacent sites to the earliest activation site at the LVS,[7] chemical ablation by ethanol infusion to the CVS,[8] and so on. Although the efficacy of radiofrequency ablation within the CVS is also limited by the distance from the coronary artery or inability to deliver adequate energy because of high impedance, ablation is highly effective if the ablation catheter is advanced to the targeted site where the anatomic distance from the coronary artery is convincingly safe. In performing anatomic approach or chemical ablation, it is important to map the CVS thoroughly including the small branches. Because the anatomic distance between the earliest activation site and the anatomically adjacent sites needs to be as close as possible for successful anatomic approach,[7] precise localization of the earliest activation site, which can be identified within the CVS branch, such as annular branch (communicating branch) or septal branch, is crucial. Identifying the true site of origin by detailed CVS mapping is also important in performing chemical ablation to decide the targeted vessel for ethanol infusion. These strategies are less invasive compared with direct epicardial ablation and always need to be prioritized before performing subxiphoid access.

SUMMARY

Direct epicardial ablation of OTVAs arising from the LVS is successful only in a minority of patients because of close proximity to the coronary artery or thick epicardial fat. Therefore, alternative strategies should be prioritized before performing epicardial approach. When performed, ECG characteristics suggestive of the site of origin to be the accessible area within the LVS needs be evaluated to avoid ineffective epicardial approach.

CLINICS CARE POINTS

- The LVS is divided into two regions: one closer to the apex of the triangle (inaccessible area), and one at the base of the triangle (accessible area).

- When the site of origin is located in the inaccessible area within the LVS, percutaneous epicardial ablation usually results in failure because of close proximity to the coronary vessels or epicardial fat.

- Preprocedural planning including evaluation of the ECG characteristics, which are useful for predicting the site of origin within the LVS, is important to avoid ineffective epicardial mapping after failed alternative ablation strategies.

DISCLOSURE

None.

REFERENCES

1. Yamada T, McElderry HT, Doppalapudi H, et al. Idiopathic ventricular arrhythmias originating from the left ventricular summit: anatomic concepts relevant to ablation. Circ Arrhythm Electrophysiol 2010;3:616–23.
2. Santangeli P, Marchlinski FE, Zado ES, et al. Percutaneous epicardial ablation of ventricular arrhythmias arising from the left ventricular summit: outcomes and electrocardiogram correlates of success. Circ Arrhythm Electrophysiol 2015;8:337–43.
3. Hayashi T, Santangeli P, Pathak RK, et al. Outcomes of catheter ablation of idiopathic outflow tract ventricular arrhythmias with an R wave pattern break in lead V2: a distinct clinical entity. J Cardiovasc Electrophysiol May 2017;28:504–14.
4. Liao H, Wei W, Tanager KS, et al. Left ventricular summit arrhythmias with an abrupt V(3) transition: anatomy of the aortic interleaflet triangle vantage point. Heart Rhythm 2021;18:10–9.
5. Chung FP, Lin CY, Shirai Y, et al. Outcomes of catheter ablation of ventricular arrhythmia originating from the left ventricular summit: a multicenter study. Heart Rhythm 2020;17:1077–83.
6. Mountantonakis SE, Frankel DS, Tschabrunn CM, et al. Ventricular arrhythmias from the coronary venous system: prevalence, mapping, and ablation. Heart Rhythm 2015;12:1145–53.
7. Shirai Y, Santangeli P, Liang JJ, et al. Anatomical proximity dictates successful ablation from adjacent sites for outflow tract ventricular arrhythmias linked to the coronary venous system. Europace 2019;21: 484–91.
8. Kreidieh B, Rodriguez-Manero M, Schurmann P, et al. Retrograde coronary venous ethanol infusion for ablation of refractory ventricular tachycardia. Circ Arrhythm Electrophysiol 2016;9:1–10.

Catheter Ablation of Left Ventricular Summit Arrhythmias from Adjacent Anatomic Vantage Points

Jorge Romero, MD, FHRS[a], Maria Gamero, MD[a], Isabella Alviz, MD[a],
Michael Grushko, MD[a], Juan Carlos Diaz, MD[a], Marta Lorente, MD[a],
Mohamed Gabr, MD[a], Cristian Camilo Toquica, MD[a], Suraj Krishnan, MD[a],
Alejandro Velasco, MD[a], Aung Lin, MD[a], Andrea Natale, MD, FHRS[b],
Fengwei Zou, MD[a], Luigi Di Biase, MD, PhD, FHRS[a],*

KEYWORDS

- Idiopathic ventricular arrhythmia • Intraventricular septum and left ventricular summit
- Cardiac ablation • Left ventricular outflow tract ventricular arrhythmia
- Epicardial mapping and ablation

KEY POINTS

- LV summit ventricular arrhythmias continue to have lower success rates of catheter ablation due to the complex anatomy of the region.
- Proper understanding of the intricate anatomy of the LV summit and novel ablation techniques can improve outcomes..

INTRODUCTION

Idiopathic ventricular arrhythmias (IVAs) originate in individuals without structural heart disease, with the majority originating from the right ventricular outflow tract (RVOT; 82%) and the remainder coming from the left ventricular outflow tract (LVOT).[1] Noteworthy, LVOT ventricular arrhythmias (VAs) can originate from different anatomic structures such as the subaortic region,[2] the coronary cusps (CC),[3] the aortic-mitral continuity (AMC), the coronary venous system,[4] and the interventricular septum (IVS) or left ventricle summit (LVS).[4–7] These multiple potential origins as well as a complex anatomic structure make LVOT VAs a challenge even for experienced electrophysiologists. It is important for the electrophysiologist in training to acquire an in-depth understanding of the regional cardiac anatomy in combination with comprehension of advanced techniques in order to increase clinical outcomes for these arrhythmias.

Catheter ablation (CA) remains the cornerstone in the modern treatment of these arrhythmias,[8] with a highly effective success rate for RVOT VAs exceeding 90%.[9] Unfortunately, CA of LVOT VAs carries a suboptimal outcome with a low success rate due to a more complex anatomic structure, reduced catheter access/mobility, catheter instability, and the presence of adjacent structures (ie, coronary arteries and epicardial fat pads) that may limit radiofrequency (RF) energy delivery.[10,11] Frequently, more than one procedure is required for long-term success.[12,13]

Interestingly, most patients with LVOT VAs are found to have several different sites with similar

[a] Montefiore Medical Center, Albert Einstein College of Medicine, Bronx, NY, USA; [b] Texas Cardiac Arrhythmia Institute, St. David's Medical Center, Austin, TX, USA
* Corresponding author. Montefiore Medical Center, Albert Einstein College of Medicine, 111 East 210th Street, Bronx, NY 10467.
E-mail address: dibbia@gmail.com

Card Electrophysiol Clin 15 (2023) 31–37
https://doi.org/10.1016/j.ccep.2022.10.001
1877-9182/23/© 2023 Elsevier Inc. All rights reserved.

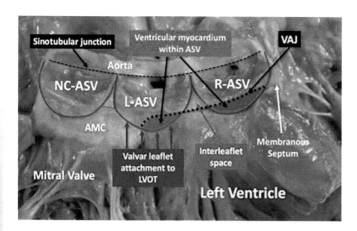

Fig. 1. Gross dissection of the LVOT anatomy showing the noncoronary aortic valve leaflet to the left. The aortic root is defined superiorly by the sinotubular junction (*black dashed line*), and inferiorly by the nadirs of the attachments of the semilunar aortic valve leaflet (*blue line*). The ventriculoarterial junction is determined by thick black dotted lines, and region where myocardium can be found in the sinus of Valsalva are showed in red. AMC, aorto-mitral continuity; NC-ASV, noncoronary aortic sinus of Valsalva; L-ASV, left aortic sinus of Valsalva; R-ASV, right aortic sinus of Valsalva; VAJ, ventriculo-arterial junction. (*From* Cheung JW, Anderson RH, Markowitz SM, Lerman BB. Catheter Ablation of Arrhythmias Originating From the Left Ventricular Outflow Tract [published correction appears in JACC Clin Electrophysiol. 2019 Apr;5(4):535]. JACC Clin Electrophysiol. 2019;5(1):1-12; with permission.)

early activation times, suggesting an intramyocardial origin of the arrhythmia, particularly in the IVS or LVS.[14–18] Different techniques have been described to address these intramyocardial foci, all associated with significant risk and suboptimal outcomes.[19] Recently, Di Biase and colleagues described an innovative technique that integrates EAM and intracardiac echocardiography (ICE) with sequential ablation of multiple early activation sites (usually shorter than −30 milliseconds pre-QRS) in LVOT VAs. Di Biase and colleagues reported an acute success rate of 93% and no recurrence in patients with successful ablation after a mean follow-up of 21 months.[20] Similar results have been demonstrated for LVS arrhythmias.[21]

Increasing knowledge, understanding, and training in the sequential CA of all early activation locations for IVS or LVS arrhythmias will improve the acute and long-term procedural outcomes. This novel method should be adopted worldwide by physicians when dealing with complex outflow tract VAs.

ANATOMY

Left Ventricular Outflow Tract and Left Ventricle Summit Anatomy

The LVOT occupies a central location in the heart, confined by the aortic root, AMC, the superior basal septum, and the LVS. The anatomic ventriculo-arterial junction marks the interface between the LV myocardial muscular aspect and the fibroelastic wall of the aortic trunk. The right aortic sinus of Valsalva forms the anterior attachment of the aorta to the LVOT, and the left aortic sinus of Valsalva forms the lateral attachment. The

posterior aspect of the LVOT abuts the left fibrous trigone and the region of the AMC. The noncoronary aortic sinus of Valsalva forms part of the AMC (**Fig. 1**).

However, the LV summit is a triangular region with its apex formed by the bifurcation of the left anterior descending (LAD) and left circumflex

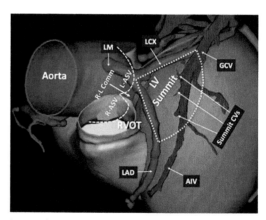

Fig. 2. The LVS is a triangular region defined by the bifurcation of the left main coronary artery forming the apex, and the first septal perforator as its base. The LVS area is demarcated with a yellow dotted line. Notice the division of the LVS by the GCV. AIV, anterior interventricular vein; GCV, great cardiac vein; LAD, left anterior descending; L-ASV, left aortic sinus of Valsalva; LCX, left circumflex; LM, left main; LV, left ventricle; R-ASV, right aortic sinus of Valsalva; R-L comm, right-left commissure; RVOT, right ventricular outflow tract. (*From* Cheung JW, Anderson RH, Markowitz SM, Lerman BB. Catheter Ablation of Arrhythmias Originating From the Left Ventricular Outflow Tract [published correction appears in JACC Clin Electrophysiol. 2019 Apr;5(4):535]. JACC Clin Electrophysiol. 2019;5(1):1-12; with permission.)

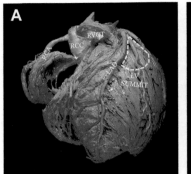
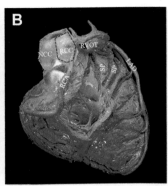
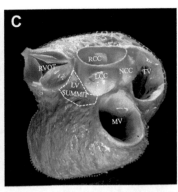

Fig. 3. LV summit anatomy (*yellow line*). (*A*) The LV summit is located at the top of the LV epicardium and is limited between the bifurcation of the LAD and the LCx coronary arteries. (*B*) The first septal perforator artery is in close relation with the LV summit (*yellow dash line*). (*C*) LV summit is in close relation with the sinuses of Valsalva (ie, LCC, RCC) and the RVOT. LAD, left anterior descending; LCC, left coronary cusp; LV, left ventricle; MV, mitral valve; NCC, noncoronary cusp; RCA, right coronary artery; RCC, right coronary cusp; RVOT, right ventricular outflow tract; SP, septal perforator; TV, tricuspid valve. (*From* Romero J, Shivkumar K, Valderrabano M, et al. Modern mapping and ablation techniques to treat ventricular arrhythmias from the left ventricular summit and interventricular septum [published correction appears in Heart Rhythm. 2020 Sep 23;:]. Heart Rhythm. 2020;17(9):1609-1620; with permission.)

arteries, and its base limited by the arc of the first septal perforator of the LAD. It is noteworthy to point out that the great cardiac vein (GCV) bisects the LVS into a superior area (anteromedial LVS on attitudinal description), which is inaccessible for epicardial CA due to its proximity to the coronary arteries along with thick epicardial fat, and an inferior area (posterolateral LVS on attitudinal description), usually a target for epicardial CA (**Fig. 2**).[22] Additionally, the LVS is in close anatomic relation with the left CC, the right coronary cusp (RCC), the RVOT, and the AMC (**Fig. 3**).

TECHNIQUE
Caveats to Electrocardiogram (ECG) Analysis for Left Ventricular Outflow Tract Arrhythmias

In general, anterior structures close to V1 will result in a left bundle branch block (LBBB) morphology. Posterior structures far from the anterior chest wall will produce a right bundle branch block (RBBB) morphology.

Considering this basic principle, RVOT VAs are usually associated with an LBBB morphology, and LVOT VAs are associated with an RBBB morphology on the electrocardiogram. However, LVOT VAs can sometimes be associated with an atypical LBBB morphology with an early precordial QRS transition (ie, at or earlier than V3). For instance, the RCC, which is immediately posterior to the septal/posterior RVOT wall, will have an LBBB pattern with early transition. Although numerous criteria have been established to help identify the possible site of

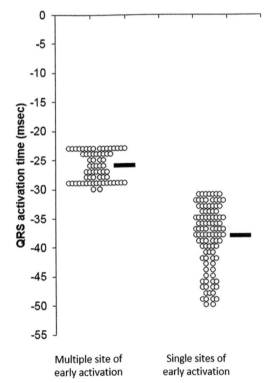

Fig. 4. Black horizontal line represents mean pre-QRS activation time. In patients with multiple early activation sites (*left panel*), the mean pre-QRS activation time was -26 ± 3 milliseconds compared with patients with a single early site (*right panel*) that was -38 ± 6 milliseconds ($P<.005$). (*From* Di Biase L, Romero J, Zado ES, et al. Variant of ventricular outflow tract ventricular arrhythmias requiring ablation from multiple sites: Intramural origin. Heart Rhythm. 2019;16(5):724-732; with permission.)

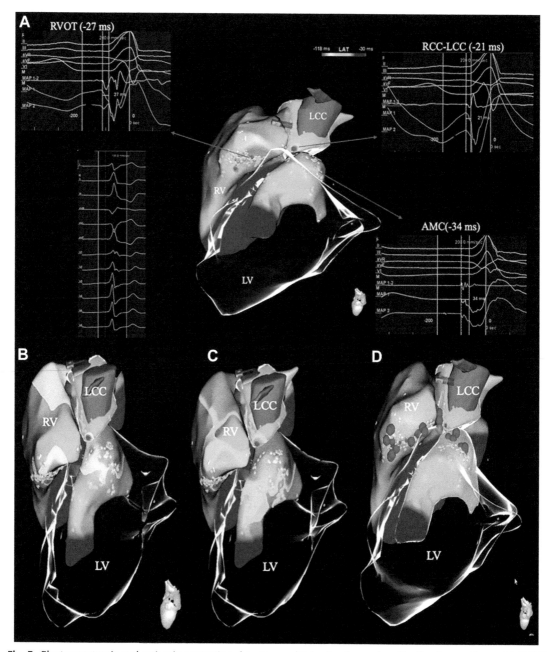

Fig. 5. Electroanatomic and activation mapping showing multiple sites for early activation in a patient with LVOT PVC. Notice similar activation times in the RVOT, RCC-LCC commissure, and AMC suggesting intramyocardial focus located in the area between these structures (LVS). AMC, aorto-mitral continuity; LCC, left coronary cusp; LV, left ventricle; RCC, right coronary cusp; RV, right ventricle. (*From* Romero J, Shivkumar K, Valderrabano M, et al. Modern mapping and ablation techniques to treat ventricular arrhythmias from the left ventricular summit and interventricular septum [published correction appears in Heart Rhythm. 2020 Sep 23;:]. Heart Rhythm. 2020;17(9):1609-1620; with permission.)

activation, ECGs are not 100% accurate identifying right versus left outflow tract origin.[5,6,23] A recent study showed that an initial QRS activation greater than 0.57 mV in the first 40 milliseconds of the QRS in lead V2 predicts an LVOT origin (accuracy 90.7%, sensitivity 84.4%, specificity 93.3%) outperforming prior ECG criteria.[24]

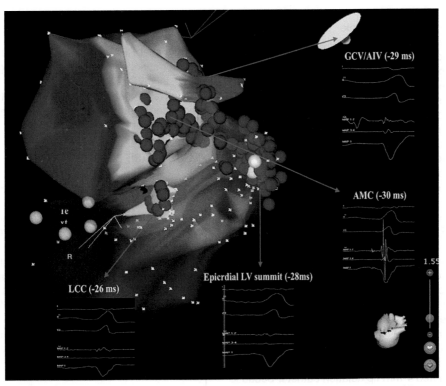

Fig. 6. Electroanatomic and activation mapping showing multiple sites of early activation. In this case, epicardial ablation was performed with modest early activation. AIV, anterior interventricular vein; AMC, aorto-mitral continuity; GCV, great cardiac vein; LCC, left coronary cusp; LV, left ventricle. (*From* Di Biase L, Romero J, Zado ES, et al. Variant of ventricular outflow tract ventricular arrhythmias requiring ablation from multiple sites: Intramural origin. Heart Rhythm. 2019;16(5):724-732; with permission.)

Electrophysiology Study and Ablation Technique

Initially, percutaneous femoral venous access and arterial access are obtained through the modified Seldinger technique using vascular ultrasound guidance. RVOT mapping is performed through the femoral venous access, LVOT mapping is performed using retrograde access via the femoral artery or through a transseptal approach. Mapping of the aortic cusps is performed using intracardiac ultrasound to confirm position and define location of the coronary artery ostia. Heparin is needed when placing catheters inside the left atrial and ventricular chambers to maintain an activating clotting time of 300 to 350 seconds. Detailed EAM of the areas of interest in the LVOT, CC, CS, and epicardium are obtained in all patients. EAM of the RVOT and epicardium is performed when needed. Activation mapping is performed to define the origin of the arrhythmia. If multiple early activation sites are found, since intramural VA/PVCs are not expected to have QS complexes, only bipolar electrograms should are used, given. After defining the earliest activation site, pace mapping is performed, though ablation should still be guided my activation mapping as it remains the

gold standard for focal VAs. Multiple early activation sites is determined using a threshold of less than 30 milliseconds pre-QRS activation time in multiple sites on activation mapping. Radiofrequency ablation (maximum power 50 W; temperature cutoff 42 C) is performed in the area displaying the earliest local electrical activation electrogram. If there are multiple early activation sites, RFA is delivered sequentially to all sites in no particular order, regardless of whether the clinical arrhythmia is suppressed from any given site. In case of manual ablation, power is uptitrated from 35W to 50W, mostly in the AMC, subaortic region, and RVOT septal wall, due to the thick nature of the myocardium, for a target impedance drop of 10 to 15% (18 ohms maximum impedance drop to avoid steam pops). It is important to emphasize the difference in the mean pre-QRS activation time between multiple early activation sites versus a single activation site (−26 ± 5 milliseconds vs −38 ±6 milliseconds; **Figs. 4 and 5**).[20] Notably, all patients with multiple early sites of activation in that study underwent epicardial mapping via subxiphoid epicardial access and/or coronary sinus cannulation.[20] Subxiphoid epicardial access is done via pericardial puncture with a 17-Tuohy epidural introducer needle under fluoroscopic guidance until ventricular pulsations are transmitted from the needle tip. Advancing the needle slightly obtains a pericardial access. Usually, a "pop" sensation with a negative pressure is felt when the needle crosses the parietal pericardium. The appearance of the cardiac silhouette marked while contrast medium is injected confirms the correct location of the needle tip. Then, a guidewire is advanced through the hollow needle projecting on multiple chambers of the heart to avoid accidental punctures of the right ventricle followed by dilatation of the puncture side of the skin with upsized dilators (5F to 8F). Afterward, an 8.5 F sheath or steerable sheath is inserted over the guidewire into the epicardial space for mapping and ablation.[25] It is important to note that endocardial as well as epicardial mapping are important to identify the origin of the VA because they frequently have an intramural focus with different exit sites (**Fig. 6**).[20]

Furthermore, it is important to highlight that patients with multiple early sites of activation with a possible intramural origin cannot be ablated using a nonirrigated 4-mm tip ablation catheter because the average lesion depth is 7.1 ± 2.6 mm, independent of duration of ablation.[26] In comparison, irrigated ablation catheters allow higher energy delivery and have shown a superior lesion depth of 9 to 13 mm, depending on ablation time.[27,28] Additionally, bipolar RF CA has been proposed as an attractive alternative using 2 ablation catheters opposed within an anatomic structure (ie, IVS) but impedance mismatch needs to be considered. Importantly, the CS, especially GCV/anterior interventricular vein (AIV) junction, will be found as one of the earliest sites in most cases. However, CA of this structure might be dangerous given the proximity with the coronary arteries in approximately 74% of the cases.[29] Therefore, a coronary angiogram needs to be performed in order to deliver RF energy in the GCV/AIV. Conversely, a recent study by Romero and colleagues demonstrated that avoiding GCV/AIV ablation has similar efficacy and safety outcomes compared with GCV/AIV ablation.[30]

LIMITATIONS

Despite the potential advantages of sequential RF CA in challenging VA such as LVOT VAs, further multicenter studies with larger samples are needed to delineate the optimal approach. Moreover, electrophysiologists in training need to be more familiar with this novel technique and gain experience with ICE epicardial and endocardial mapping.

SUMMARY

A sequential RF CA technique should be considered in patient with multiple sites of origin, particularly in LVOT VAs such as LVS VAs. The innovative CA technique described in this review article demonstrates a high success rate acutely and at time of follow-up.

CLINICS CARE POINTS

- The use of ICE and EAM for endocardial and epicardial can facilitate and improve outcomes for LV summit ablation.
- Ventricular arrhythmias with multiple activation sites, defined as multiple early sites with pre-QRS activation time <30 ms, can be targeted through sequential ablation of all the early activation sites.
- Irrigated catheter tips allow for higher lesion depth, which may be necessary in ablation of VAs with multiple early activation sites and possible intramural origin.

DISCLOSURE

Dr L. Di Biase is a consultant for Stereotaxis, Biosense Webster, Boston Scientific, Abbott Medical and has received speaker honoraria/travel from Medtronic, Atricure, Bristol Meyers Squibb, Pfizer, and Biotronik. Dr A. Natale is a consultant for Biosense Webster, Stereotaxis, Abbott and has received speaker honoraria/travel from Medtronic, Atricure, Biotronik, and Janssen. The remaining authors report no conflict of interest.

REFERENCES

1. Iwai S, Cantillon DJ, Kim RJ, et al. Right and left ventricular outflow tract tachycardias: evidence for a common electrophysiologic mechanism. J Cardiovasc Electrophysiol 2006;17:1052–8.
2. Callans DJ, Menz V, Schwartzman D, et al. Repetitive monomorphic tachycardia from the left ventricular outflow tract: electrocardiographic patterns consistent with a left ventricular site of origin. J Am Coll Cardiol 1997;29:1023–7.
3. Ouyang F, Fotuhi P, Ho SY, et al. Repetitive monomorphic ventricular tachycardia originating from the aortic sinus cusp: electrocardiographic characterization for guiding catheter ablation. J Am Coll Cardiol 2002;39:500–8.
4. Daniels DV, Lu YY, Morton JB, et al. Idiopathic epicardial left ventricular tachycardia originating remote from the sinus of Valsalva:

electrophysiological characteristics, catheter abla-tion, and identification from the 12-lead electrocar-diogram. Circulation 2006;113:1659–66.

5. Obel OA. d'Avila A, Neuzil P, Saad EB, Ruskin JN, Reddy VY. Ablation of left ventricular epicardial outflow tract tachycardia from the distal great car-diac vein. J Am Coll Cardiol 2006;48:1813–7.

6. Tada H, Nogami A, Naito S, et al. Left ventricular epicardial outflow tract tachycardia: a new distinct subgroup of outflow tract tachycardia. Jpn Circ J 2001;65:723–30.

7. Ito S, Tada H, Naito S, et al. Simultaneous mapping in the left sinus of valsalva and coronary venous sys-tem predicts successful catheter ablation from the left sinus of valsalva. Pacing Clin Electrophysiol 2005;28(Suppl 1):S150–4.

8. Hayashi T, Liang JJ, Shirai Y, et al. Trends in suc-cessful ablation sites and outcomes of ablation for idiopathic outflow tract ventricular arrhythmias. JACC Clin Electrophysiol 2020;6(2):221–30.

9. Kim RJ, Iwai S, Markowitz SM, et al. Clinical and electro-physiological spectrum of idiopathic ventricular outflow tract arrhythmias. J Am Coll Cardiol 2007;49:2035–43.

10. Schweikert RA, Saliba WI, Tomassoni G, et al. Percu-taneous pericardial instrumentation for endo-epicardial mapping of previously failed ablations. Circulation 2003;108:1329–35.

11. Latchamsetty R, Yokokawa M, Morady F, et al. Multi-center outcomes for catheter ablation of idiopathic Premature ventricular complexes. JACC Clin Elec-trophysiol 2015;1(3):116–23.

12. Coggins DL, Lee RJ, Sweeney J, et al. Radiofre-quency catheter ablation as a cure for idiopathic tachycardia of both left and right ventricular origin. J Am Coll Cardiol 1994;23:1333–41.

13. Ito S, Tada H, Naito S, et al. Development and vali-dation of an ECG algorithm for identifying the optimal ablation site for idiopathic ventricular outflow tract tachycardia. J Cardiovasc Electrophysiol 2003; 14:1280–6.

14. Yamada T, Maddox WR, McElderry HT, et al. Radio-frequency catheter ablation of idiopathic ventricular arrhythmias originating from intramural foci in the left ventricular outflow tract: efficacy of sequential versus simultaneous unipolar catheter ablation. Circ Arrhythm Electrophysiol 2015;8:344–52.

15. Teh AW, Reddy VY, Koruth JS, et al. Bipolar radiofre-quency catheter ablation for refractory ventricular outflow tract arrhythmias. J Cardiovasc Electrophy-siol 2014;25:1093–9.

16. Tholakanahalli VN, Bertog S, Roukoz H, et al. Cath-eter ablation of ventricular tachycardia using intra-coronary wire mapping and coil embolization: description of a new technique. Heart Rhythm 2013;10:292–6.

17. Baher A, Shah DJ, Valderrabano M. Coronary venous ethanol infusion for the treatment of refractory ventricular tachycardia. Heart Rhythm 2012;9:1637–9.

18. Sapp JL, Beeckler C, Pike R, et al. Initial human feasibility of infusion needle catheter ablation for re-fractory ventricular tachycardia. Circulation 2013; 128:2289–95.

19. Lavalle C, Mariani MV, Piro A, et al. Electrocardio-graphic features, mapping and ablation of idiopathic outflow tract ventricular arrhythmias. J Interv Card Electrophysiol 2020;57(2):207–18.

20. Di Biase L, Romero J, Zado ES, et al. Variant of ven-tricular outflow tract ventricular arrhythmias requiring ablation from multiple sites: intramural origin. Heart Rhythm 2019;16:724–32.

21. Romero J, Shivkumar K, Valderrabano M, et al. Mod-ern mapping and ablation techniques to treat ven-tricular arrhythmias from the left ventricular summit and interventricular septum. Heart Rhythm 2020; 17(9):1609–20.

22. Cheung JW, Anderson RH, Markowitz SM, et al. Catheter ablation of arrhythmias originating from the left ventricular outflow tract. JACC Clin Electro-physiol 2019;5(1):1–12.

23. Tanner H, Hindricks G, Schirdewahn P, et al. Outflow tract tachycardia with R/S transition in lead V3: Six different anatomic approaches for successful abla-tion. J Am Coll Cardiol 2005;45:418–23.

24. Xia Y, Liu Z, Liu J, et al. Amplitude of QRS complex within initial 40 ms in V2 (V2QRSi40): Novel electro-cardiographic criterion for predicting accurate local-ization of outflow tract ventricular arrhythmia origin. Heart Rhythm 2020;17(12):2164–71.

25. Sosa E, Scanavacca M, d'Avila A, et al. A new tech-nique to perform epicardial mapping in the electro-physiology laboratory. J Cardiovasc Electrophysiol 1996;7:531–6.

26. Simmers TA, Wittkampf FH, Hauer RN, et al. In vivo ventricular lesion growth in radiofrequency catheter ablation. Pacing Clin Electrophysiol PACE 1994;17: 523–31.

27. Ruffy R, Imran MA, Santel DJ, et al. Radiofrequency delivery through a cooled catheter tip allows the cre-ation of larger endomyocardial lesions in the ovine heart. J Cardiovasc Electrophysiol 1995;6:1089–96.

28. Callans DJ, Ren JF, Narula N, et al. Effects of linear, irrigated-tip radiofrequency ablation in porcine healed anterior infarction. J Cardiovasc Electrophy-siol 2001;12:1037–42.

29. Nagashima K, Choi EK, Lin KY, et al. Ventricular ar-rhythmias near the distal great cardiac vein: chal-lenging arrhythmia for ablation. Circ A&e 2014;7: 906–12.

30. Romero J, Velasco A, Diaz JC, et al. Fluoroless versus conventional mapping and ablation of ven-tricular arrhythmias arising from the left ventricular summit and interventricular septum. Circ Arrhythmia Electrophysiol 2022 Jul;15(7):e010547.

Intramyocardial Mapping of Ventricular Arrhythmias via Septal Venous Perforators
Defining the Superior Intraseptal Space

Gustavo S. Guandalini, MD

KEYWORDS

- Basal superior intraseptal • Catheter ablation • Coronary venous mapping • Left ventricular summit
- Premature ventricular contractions

KEY POINTS

- A significant proportion of outflow tract arrhythmias has an intramyocardial site of origin, accessible for mapping from intraseptal perforator veins, and termed the basal superior intraseptal space.
- This additional mapping is important to differentiate from those originating from the true epicardial surface of the left ventricular summit when endocardial mapping and ablation fails.
- The basal superior intraseptal arrhythmias can often be targeted from the endocardium, even from anatomic vantage points that otherwise fail to demonstrate presystolic activation.
- Intramyocardial mapping for arrhythmias suspected to originate from the left ventricular summit can have a positive impact on acute procedural success.

INTRODUCTION

The left ventricular summit (LVS), as originally described by McAlpine, refers to the highest point of the LV epicardium, where the upper end of the anterior interventricular sulcus joins the aortic portion of the LV ostium.[1] This anatomic location has become increasingly recognized as an important source for ventricular arrhythmias, often quoted as the presumed site of origin when mapping endocardial outflow tract structures, as well as the right and left sinuses of Valsalva of the aortic valve, fails to demonstrate the site of origin with activation or pace mapping. Such finding implies an epicardial site of origin that is inaccessible from the endocardial right ventricular outflow tract (RVOT) and left ventricular outflow tract (LVOT), justifying procedural failure when endocardial-only mapping and ablation is performed.

Demonstration of a true epicardial origin from the LVS can be achieved either by coronary venous mapping from the anterior interventricular vein (AIV) or via direct percutaneous epicardial mapping. In both instances, however, successful ablation remains challenging because of (1) anatomical constraints preventing proper placement of the ablation catheter beyond the great cardiac vein (GCV) into the AIV, (2) inadequate radiofrequency current delivery due to high impedance, (3) proximity to coronary arteries with risk of myocardial infarction from direct coronary injury during ablation, and (4) the presence of epicardial fat covering the atrioventricular annulus, preventing lesion formation on the epicardial surface of the LVS when percutaneous epicardial access is performed.[2,3]

In addition to a true epicardial site of origin, another challenge to map and ablate outflow tract ventricular arrhythmias refers to intramural

The author has no conflicts to disclose.
Section of Cardiac Electrophysiology, Hospital of the University of Pennsylvania – Pavilion, One Convention Avenue, Level 2 – City Side, Philadelphia, PA 19104, USA
E-mail address: Gustavo.Guandalini@pennmedicine.upenn.edu

Card Electrophysiol Clin 15 (2023) 39–47
https://doi.org/10.1016/j.ccep.2022.10.004
1877-9182/23/Published by Elsevier Inc.

sources. Even though microelectrode catheters have long been used for epicardial mapping via the coronary venous circulation to preclude the need for percutaneous epicardial access,[4] intramyocardial mapping for LVS arrhythmias was first reported only over a decade later. This was performed from a septal perforating branch of the AIV, with this intraseptal recording revealing the earliest activation with perfect pace map after both endocardial and epicardial mapping from the AIV failed to reveal the true site of origin.[5] Despite being described as a procedural failure due to inability to advance the ablation catheter into this small tributary of the AIV, this very observation led to subsequent reports of intramyocardial mapping for LVS arrhythmias,[6–8] which in turn resulted in larger series showing successful ablation from adjacent structures and anatomically guided by this tridimensional mapping of the intramyocardial aspect of the LVS.[9–12]

Definitions: Basal Superior Intraseptal Versus Epicardial Left Ventricular Summit

Although any non-endocardial site of origin for outflow tract ventricular arrhythmias has traditionally been labeled as originating from the *LVS*, systematic intramyocardial mapping helped distinguish a true *epicardial* LVS site or origin from those originating from the intramyocardial aspect of the outflow tract, in turn named the *basal superior intraseptal* (SIS) space.[13] Such systematic approach is important to bring clarity to these anatomic definitions and can impact procedural success. A significant proportion of patients who undergo intraseptal mapping from septal

venous perforator branches of the AIV show presystolic activation from the SIS space. In such instances, in which the site of origin is deemed intraseptal, successful endocardial ablation can be achieved in a significant minority of cases despite failing to demonstrate presystolic endocardial activation. These observations can be best illustrated with the case studies described below.

Case study 1: Superior intraseptal origin with presystolic endocardial activation and successful endocardial ablation

History. A 58-year-old man with high-burden (41%), symptomatic premature ventricular contractions (PVCs) that failed two prior ablations (both limited to the RVOT) and antiarrhythmic drugs (flecainide and propafenone) was referred for repeat ablation. Clinical electrocardiogram (ECG) showed frequent PVCs in bigeminy, with left bundle right inferior axis and V2 transition, highly suggestive of LVOT site of origin and explaining prior procedural failure at the referring institution (**Fig. 1**, left).

Intraprocedural findings. Intraprocedurally, ECG recording of the PVC suggested later transition compared with the clinical ECG (V4 transition, see **Fig. 1**, right), so the RVOT was mapped first. The site of earliest activation was the anterior aspect of the septal RVOT (35 ms pre-QRS), but the signal at this site suggested far-field recording (although previously ablated) and pace-mapping from this site was also poor (wider QRS with later transition and positive QRS complex in lead I, **Fig. 2**). Epicardial mapping from the AIV was pursued next, in

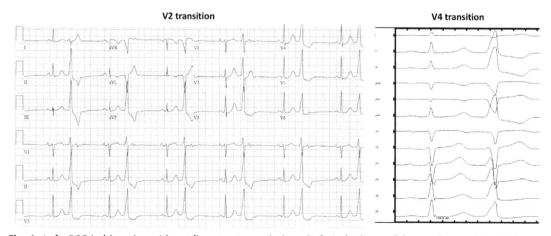

Fig. 1. Left: ECG in bigeminy with outflow tract morphology (inferiorly directed) but early transition (V2), suggestive of LVOT rather than RVOT site of origin. Right: Intraprocedural ECG showed right inferior axis but with later transition (V4, although still earlier than sinus), suggestive of septal anterior RVOT site of origin despite two prior ablations from this site at the referring institution.

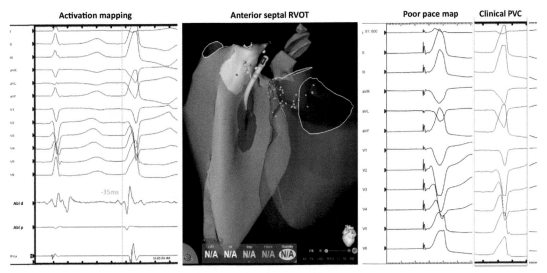

Fig. 2. Left: Activation mapping from anterior septal RVOT showing far-field, presystolic activation (35 ms pre-QRS). Middle: Electroanatomic map showing catheter position at the site of earliest activation (opposite to right coronary cusp in *purple*). Right: Pace mapping from the same site, showing poor match with wider QRS, later transition and positive deflection in lead I. (*From* Nakatani Y, Vlachos K, Ramirez FD, et al. Acute coronary artery occlusion and ischemia-related ventricular tachycardia during catheter ablation in the right ventricular outflow tract. J Cardiovasc Electrophysiol. 2021;32(2):547-550. doi:10.1111/jce.14809.)

anticipation for LVOT mapping afterward. However, when placing a 4Fr decapolar mapping catheter from the coronary sinus into the AIV (Map-iT, Access Point Technologies, Minneapolis, MN), its tip landed in a septal branch of the AIV, revealing intraseptal recordings from the SIS space (**Fig. 3**). Interestingly, this site showed not only presystolic activation (37 ms pre-QRS) with sharp electrograms (suggestive of local rather than far-field recording), but also excellent pace map (95% match) from its distal bipole (**Fig. 4**). Although suggestive of SIS site of origin, LVOT mapping had to be completed before determining this to have true intraseptal source. This was performed via retroaortic approach, including the aortic valve cusps and the endocardial LVOT. The site of earliest activation was the LVOT below the right coronary cusp, with activation 22 ms pre-QRS that was later than that of the SIS mapping (**Fig. 5**). Still, catheter in this location led to mechanical suppression of the PVC, so ablation was performed with suppression after less than 10 seconds (**Fig. 6**) with no recurrence.

Summary. In this case, there was clear demonstration of an SIS site of origin for the clinical PVC, which also explained the far-field presystolic activation from the RVOT that led to two prior failed ablations. However, there was also clear presystolic activation from the endocardial LVOT from where the PVC was successfully eliminated, which raises the question of the true utility of performing SIS mapping. If a clear target could be found endocardially, was the extra effort to map the intraseptal space an academically interesting but practically irrelevant one?

Case study 2: Superior intraseptal origin without presystolic endocardial activation, yet successfully ablated endocardially

History. A 52-year-old woman with symptomatic PVCs and non-sustained ventricular tachycardia (NSVT) for several years (**Fig. 7**) with concomitant cardiomyopathy (Ejection fraction (EF) 40%) was referred for repeat ablation after failing antiarrhythmic drugs (sotalol) and two prior ablations, one of which complicated with complete heart block leading to biventricular pacemaker implantation.

Intraprocedural findings. As this patient failed prior extensive ablation from both RVOT and LVOT, decision was made to map the SIS space upfront to determine if an intraseptal origin was the reason for failure. A coronary venogram was performed (**Fig. 8**, left), showing a small intraseptal branch of the AIV that was selectively engaged with a 4Fr hydrophilic sheath (see **Fig. 8**, center) from which a 2Fr octapolar microcatheter (EPStar, Baylis Medical, Mississauga, ON) was delivered to the SIS space (see **Fig. 8**, right). This site revealed not only presystolic activation (22 ms pre-QRS) but also excellent pace map (98.4% match), all suggestive of an intramural source for the clinical

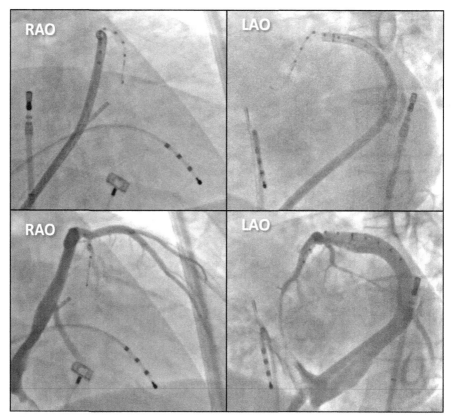

Fig. 3. Top: Fluoroscopic position of a 4Fr decapolar catheter with its proximal portion in the AIV, but its tip diving toward the interventricular septum. Bottom: Coronary venography confirms catheter placement in a rather large proximal septal branch of the AIV, revealing the *superior intraseptal* space.

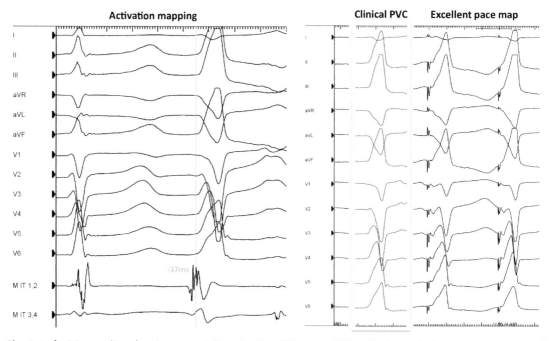

Fig. 4. Left: SIS recording showing presystolic activation (37 ms pre-QRS) with sharp electrograms, suggestive of near-field recording with possible intraseptal site of origin. Right: Pace map from the same location showing 95% match (clinical PVC highlighted for comparison), with negative QRS deflection in lead I compared with that obtained from the septal RVOT.

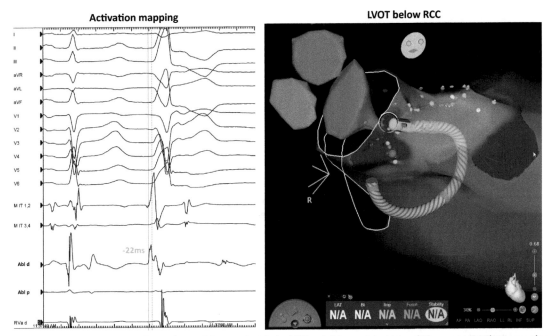

Fig. 5. Left: Best activation from the LVOT recorded below the right coronary cusp (22 ms pre-QRS). Decapolar catheter previously placed in the septal branch of the AIV lost its original distal position, but still earlier than the ablator electrogram (*continuous line*).

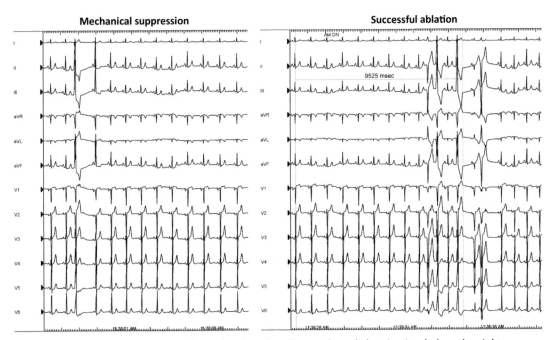

Fig. 6. Left: Mechanical suppression from the site of earliest endocardial activation below the right coronary cusp. Right: Successful ablation from the endocardial LVOT below the right coronary cusp, with relatively late suppression after approximately 10 seconds from ablation onset. The last PVC recorded is superiorly directed (nonclinical).

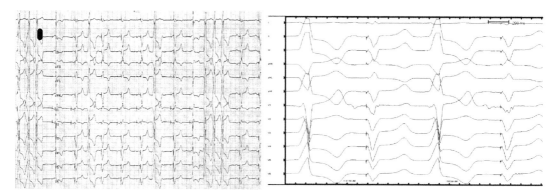

Fig. 7. Clinical ECG showing frequent PVCs and NSVT with left bundle, right inferior axis, and abrupt V3 transition, with underlying sinus rhythm with biventricular-paced rhythm due to iatrogenic complete heart block.

PVC (**Fig. 9**). Extensive mapping from neighboring structures was accomplished, none of which showed better activation or pace maps: 11 ms pre-QRS from septal RVOT with poor pace map, 9 ms pre-QRS from septal pulmonic cusp although with excellent pace map (97.6% match), on time epicardial activation from AIV, 10 ms post-QRS from left coronary cusp, and on time endocardial activation from the junction of the right and left coronary cusps below the aortic valve, which was the best LVOT activation obtained and in closest proximity to the intraseptal microcatheter (**Fig. 10**, left and center). Despite no presystolic

activation from the right-left junction, ablation from this vantage point led to nearly immediate PVC suppression without recurrence (see **Fig. 10**, right).

Summary. Similar to the prior case, the site of origin was also the SIS space, with earliest activation and best pace map despite very extensive mapping of all neighboring structures. In contrast, however, the site of successful ablation did not demonstrate presystolic activation and was attempted solely based on anatomic proximity. In the following section, the authors discuss how often this is the case, which quantifies the true

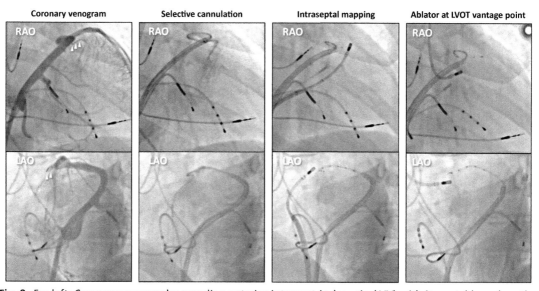

Fig. 8. Far left: Coronary venography revealing anterior interventricular vein (AIV) with its septal branches; the most basal is marked (*white arrows*). Center left: most proximal septal branch from the AIV selectively cannulated with 4Fr sheath, with selective venogram performed showing intraseptal course from this branch. Center right: 2Fr octapolar catheter placed intraseptally from the previously deployed 4Fr sheath, with ablator in opposite position from most anterior aspect of the septal right ventricular outflow tract. Far right: Ablator in closest anatomic vantage point on the LVOT, below the right-left junction and from where successful ablation was performed.

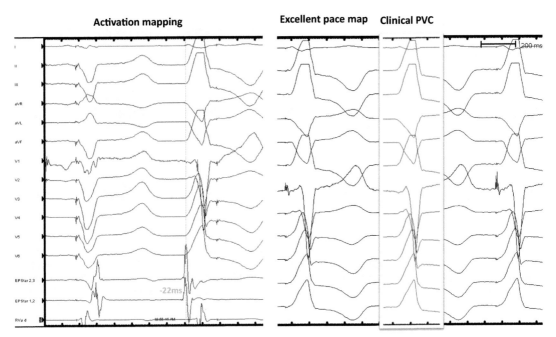

Fig. 9. Intraseptal activation showing pre-QRS electrograms (22 ms pre-QRS from EPStar 1,2) and excellent pace map (98.4% match).

impact of SIS mapping as these would otherwise likely result in acute procedural failure.

DISCUSSION

When LVOT arrhythmias fail to be eliminated from the endocardium despite adequate mapping and ablation, a *left ventricular summit* site of origin is often suspected. Although this is true for a proportion of cases, mapping and ablating from the AIV often fails to confirm an epicardial origin in such cases. This in turn is frequently attributed to mapping an entire surface only from the anatomic constraints of the AIV itself, which fits an *endocardial versus epicardial* paradigm for approaching these outflow tract arrhythmias. In addition, although AIV mapping can be relatively easily performed with current mapping catheters, ablation from this site can be rather challenging, among other

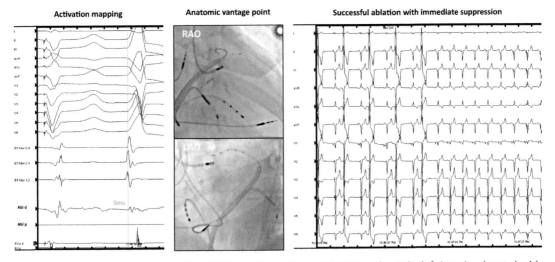

Fig. 10. Despite no presystolic activation (*left*) from the endocardial LVOT at the right-left junction (*center*), ablation from this vantage point in close proximity to the intraseptal source led to nearly immediate PVC suppression (*right*).

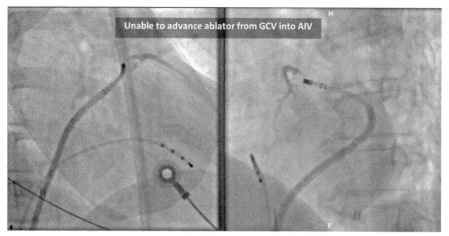

Fig. 11. Example of anatomic constraints precluding epicardial ablation via the anterior interventricular vein due to inability to advance the catheter beyond the great cardiac vein. A deflectable sheath is placed distally in the coronary sinus toward the great cardiac vein, and the ablation catheter is advanced as distal as possible in the great cardiac vein but unable to turn anteriorly toward the anterior interventricular vein. A selective venogram is performed by injecting contrast through the ablation catheter itself, confirming the difficulty to accommodate this catheter into a smaller venous target. Left, right anterior oblique view; right, left anterior oblique view.

issues due to difficulty advancing the ablation catheter beyond the GCV into the AIV (**Fig. 11**).

A number of strategies have been developed to overcome these challenges in ablating non-endocardial outflow tract arrhythmias, all expertly described in this edition of the *Left Ventricular Summit Electrophysiology Clinics*. These include endocardial ablation from vantage points to approximate the presumed site of origin, employment of bipolar ablation, chemical ablation with ethanol injection from intraseptal venous branches, and even surgical dissection of the epicardial fat for direct epicardial radiofrequency ablation. The implication from the success observed with some of these strategies, however, is the recognition of an intramyocardial source for these arrhythmias, such that ablation from adjacent sites that otherwise would not predict arrhythmia suppression (due to poor activation or pace mapping) leads to successful ablation.

Therefore, the current paradigm for mapping and ablating outflow tract arrhythmias should incorporate the *basal SIS* space as the intramyocardial region between the endocardial outflow tract and the epicardial surface of the LVS. Such tridimensional mapping not only helps better understand their true site of origin but also explains the ability to successfully ablate from vantage points without presystolic activation, as described by the second case study. A puzzling observation then relates to the fact that activation times can be significantly different despite close anatomic proximity. This probably reflects preferential anisotropic myocardial conduction, such that depolarization wavefronts exhibit faster conduction parallel to myocardial fiber orientation—explaining the high proportion of presystolic SIS activation even if the septal branch of the AIV is not exactly within the true intramural source—compared with perpendicular conduction across different fibers—explaining postsystolic activation from the endocardium despite being in close proximity to the intramural source.

The remaining issue then is how often is SIS origin found in outflow tract arrhythmias and what is the actual impact of SIS mapping in acute procedural success. In a case series of patients who underwent SIS mapping with a unipolar mapping wire, 45.5% of patients (20 out of 44) exhibited SIS origin, defined as the earliest activation site after mapping neighboring structures. Of these, 50% (10 out of 20) also showed presystolic activation from the endocardial LVOT and were successfully ablated from these sites (similar to Case Study 1). Another 10% (2 out of 20) showed presystolic activation from the epicardial LVS and were successfully ablated from the AIV, whereas 15% (3 out of 20) had acute procedural failure. Importantly, 25% of those with SIS origin (5 out of 20 or 11.3% of all 44 patients in this series) were successfully ablated endocardially despite no presystolic endocardial activation (similar to Case Study 2), which represents the proportion of patients who would otherwise exhibit procedural failure if not for mapping the basal SIS space.[13] Although this is a highly selected population with significant referral bias after failed procedures, this is the best estimate of the true impact of this approach after systematic SIS mapping in a series of patients with suspected LVS arrhythmias.

SUMMARY

In this article, the authors described a distinct intramyocardial region in the LVOT named the *basal superior intraseptal* space. Although this is not accessible for direct ablation, mapping from this region can be achieved from septal perforators from the AIV. Almost half of patients suspected to have LVS arrhythmias exhibit SIS origin. A significant minority of patients (approximately 10%) can be successfully ablated from endocardial sites without presystolic activation, targeting from vantage points in close proximity to the site of origin. Therefore, this additional step in mapping LVS arrhythmias not only expands our understanding of their true sites of origin but can also improve procedural success in these rather challenging scenarios.

FUNDING

Mark Marchlinski EP Research and Education Fund.

CLINICS CARE POINTS

- A significant proportion of outflow tract arrhythmias has an intramyocardial site of origin, accessible for mapping from intraseptal perforator veins, and termed the *basal superior intraseptal space.*
- This additional mapping is important to differentiate from those originating from the true *epicardial* surface of the *left ventricular summit* when endocardial mapping and ablation fails.
- The *basal superior intraseptal* arrhythmias can often be targeted from the endocardium, even from anatomic vantage points that otherwise fail to demonstrate presystolic activation.
- Intramyocardial mapping for arrhythmias suspected to originate from the left ventricular summit can have a positive impact on acute procedural success.

REFERENCES

1. McAlpine WA. Heart and coronary arteries: an anatomical atlas for clinical diagnosis, radiological investigation, and surgical treatment. New York: Springer-Verlag; 1977.
2. Nagashima K, Choi E-K, Lin KY, et al. Ventricular arrhythmias near the distal great cardiac vein: challenging arrhythmia for ablation. Circ Arrhythm Electrophysiol 2014;7(5):906–12.
3. Enriquez A, Malavassi F, Saenz LC, et al. How to map and ablate left ventricular summit arrhythmias. Heart Rhythm 2017;14(1):141–8.
4. de Paola AA, Melo WD, Távora MZ, et al. Angiographic and electrophysiological substrates for ventricular tachycardia mapping through the coronary veins. Heart 1998;79(1):59–63.
5. Yamada T, Okada T, Murakami Y, et al. Premature ventricular contractions arising from the intramural ventricular septum. Pacing Clin Electrophysiol 2009;32:e1–3.
6. Yokokawa M, Good E, Chugh A, et al. Intramural idiopathic ventricular arrhythmias originating in the intraventricular septum. Circ Arrhythm Electrophysiol 2012;5:258–63.
7. Chen H, Shehata M, Swerdlow C, et al. Intramural outflow tract ventricular tachycardia. Circ Arrhythm Electrophysiol 2014;7:978–81.
8. Yamada T, Doppalapudi H, Maddox WR, et al. Prevalence and electrocardiographic and electrophysiological characteristics of idiopathic ventricular arrhythmias originating from intramural foci in the left ventricular outflow tract. Circ Arrhythm Electrophysiol 2016;9:e004079.
9. Komatsu Y, Nogami A, Shinoda Y, et al. Idiopathic ventricular arrhythmias originating from the vicinity of the communicating vein of cardiac venous systems at the left ventricular summit. Circ Arrhythm Electrophysiol 2018;11(1):e005386.
10. Ghannam M, Liang J, Sharaf-Dabbagh G, et al. Mapping and ablation of intramural ventricular arrhythmias: a stepwise approach focused on the site of origin. JACC Clin Electrophysiol 2020;6(11):1339–48.
11. Tavares L, Lador A, Fuentes S, et al. Intramural venous ethanol infusion for refractory ventricular arrhythmias: outcomes of a multicenter experience. JACC Clin Electrophysiol 2020;6(11):1420–31.
12. Liao H, Wei W, Tanager KS, et al. Left ventricular summit arrhythmias with an abrupt V3 transition: anatomy of the aortic interleaflet triangle vantage point. Heart Rhythm 2021;18(1):10–9.
13. Guandalini GS, Santangeli P, Schaller R, et al. Intramyocardial mapping of ventricular premature depolarizations via septal venous perforators: differentiating the superior intraseptal region from left ventricular summit origins. Heart Rhythm 2022;19(9):1475–83.

Ablation of Focal Intramural Outflow Tract Ventricular Arrhythmias

Jackson J. Liang, DO, Frank Bogun, MD*

KEYWORDS

• Intramural • Ablation • Ventricular arrhythmia • PVC • Ventricular tachycardia

KEY POINTS

• Intramural OT VAs can be challenging to eliminate with catheter ablation
• CMR can help to exclude occult scar and nonischemic cardiomyopathy in patients with intramural OT VAs
• Identification of the true site of origin can facilitate successful ablation of intramural VAs

INTRODUCTION

Catheter ablation is an effective and increasingly used treatment of focal ventricular arrhythmias (VAs). Most idiopathic VAs originate from the outflow tract (OT) region and can be targeted with ablation from the endocardial aspect of the right ventricular (RV) and left ventricular (LV) OTs, or from above or below the aortic sinuses of Valsalva (ASV).[1,2] However, in some patients with OT VAs, the true site of origin (SOO) may have an intramural in origin,[3] either from the septal OT, or from the anterior LV ostium (ie, LV summit region). Ablation of intramural OT VAs is often challenging due to difficulties with mapping to identify the true SOO, as well as reaching the true SOO with ablation due to an intramural location. Because branches of the coronary venous system (CVS) often course through the midmyocardial aspect of the LV anteroseptum and LV summit region, the CVS can serve as an anatomic access point to permit mapping and ablation of intramural OT VAs.[4]

IDENTIFICATION AND SIGNIFICANCE OF INTRAMURAL SCAR

In patients with OT VAs and normal LV ejection function with apparently structurally normal hearts on transthoracic echocardiography, it is important to rule out the presence of underlying scar and occult nonischemic cardiomyopathy (NICM). Cardiac delayed enhancement magnetic resonance (CMR) imaging has been shown to be helpful to identify the presence of scar and localize the SOO and critical VA substrates in patients with NICM.[5]

CMR should be considered in patients with frequent VAs as the presence of scar on CMR may identify occult NICM and can be associated with increased long-term risk of sudden death. All patients with scar on CMR and newly diagnosed NICM should undergo programmed ventricular stimulation at the time of the ablation procedure to assess for long-term risk of sudden death. Ghannam and colleagues previously performed delayed enhancement CMR in 272 patients with normal LV function undergoing ablation of apparently idiopathic VAs and scarring was identified in 67 (25%) of these patients. All patients underwent VA ablation with programmed ventricular stimulation at the time of the procedure. There were 7 (3%) patients with inducible sustained VT and during long-term follow-up, and inducibility for sustained VA had 71% positive predictive value and 100% negative predictive value to predict recurrence of VA during follow-up.[6]

Electrophysiology Section, Division of Cardiovascular Medicine, Department of Internal Medicine, University of Michigan, Ann Arbor, MI, USA
* Corresponding author. Cardiovascular Center, University of Michigan Medical Center, Ann Arbor, MI 48104.
E-mail address: fbogun@med.umich.edu

Card Electrophysiol Clin 15 (2023) 49–56
https://doi.org/10.1016/j.ccep.2022.04.006
1877-9182/23/© 2023 Elsevier Inc. All rights reserved.

Importantly, the underlying CMR scar pattern can be predictive of long-term sudden death risk, and one large multicenter study by Muser and colleagues[7] has demonstrated that the presence of a ring-like pattern of delayed enhancement to be associated with a particularly high risk of developing sustained VAs.

In addition, identification of intramural scar is helpful because it can help to localize possible ablation sites and predict ablation outcome. We previously examined 56 patients with intramural VAs who underwent CMR before VA ablation, in whom ablation was successful in 75%. We found that ablation was more likely to be successful in those patients whose scar was more superficial to the endocardium. Furthermore, change in the VA morphology was occasionally seen in 32% of patients during breakout site ablation, and further ablation targeting a different site within the scar resulted in successful elimination of VA the majority (75%) of the time.[8] We have also recently shown the value of CMR for identifying the presence of peri-aortic scar and to define the location and the extent of scarring, which may be targeted with ablation from above the ASV in some patients with OT VAs and NICM.[9]

Importantly, there is a small subset of patients in whom CMR may miss the presence of septal VA substrate and scar, which can be detected with invasive voltage mapping.[10] The quality of CMR images may be variable between patients and centers, especially in patients with cardiac implantable electronic devices (CIED). Artifacts due to the CIED generator or leads may impair the diagnostic value of CMR and artifact reducing CMR sequences with broadband image acquisition should be performed.[11] Briceño and colleagues showed that among patients with suspected intramural VA originating within the interventricular septum, mapping of the septal coronary veins can be helpful to identify the presence of scar, which may represent VA substrate. Wire-mapping of the septal perforator branches of the AIV in these patients with NICM and VAs originating from within the septum to be a helpful strategy to identify low-voltage fractionated unipolar electrograms, which could represent VA substrate worth targeting with ablation.[12]

OUR APPROACH TO PREPROCEDURAL EVALUATION, MAPPING, AND ABLATION OF INTRAMURAL OUTFLOW TRACT VENTRICULAR ARRHYTHMIAS
Preprocedure Evaluation

All patients undergo transthoracic echocardiogram to assess cardiac function and dimensions.

Outpatient event monitoring including ambulatory 12-lead Holter monitoring is performed to evaluate VA burden and morphology. In patients with high (>10%) premature ventricular complex (PVC) burden or other high-risk features such as the presence of multiple PVC morphologies, documented nonsustained or sustained VT, presyncope or presyncope, stress testing, and cardiac MRI should be performed to assess for the presence of scar and structural heart disease. Age and LV ejection fraction have also been demonstrated to predict the likelihood of scar on CMR.[13] Cardiac computed tomography angiography (CTA) is often performed as well before ablation, with focus on the anatomic course of the coronary arteries and veins. Specifically, cardiac CTA can assist in visualizing the course of the septal branches of the CVS, which may be used to facilitate mapping and ablation of intramural OT VAs. The cardiac anatomy and CMR scar can be registered using the MUSIC software, which permits integration into the map created with 3D electroanatomic mapping at the time of the procedure.

Mapping of the right ventricular and left ventricular Outflow Tracts

No clear ECG characteristics have been identified to definitively indicate an intramural origin of VAs. In patients with suspected intramural OT VAs, all chambers are mapped before ablation to identify the earliest activation sites and best pace-maps for the clinical VA. Typically, the septal RV and right ventricular outflow tract (RVOT) are mapped first using an ablation catheter through a fixed (SR-0; Abbott, Chicago, IL) or steerable sheath (Agilis; Abbott, Chicago, IL). For LV anteroseptal and LV summit PVCs, femoral arterial access is also obtained for retrograde mapping of the ASV and the LV endocardium below the aortic valve, as well as to facilitate coronary angiography if needed. Specifically, detailed activation and pace-mapping of the region above and below the right ASV, left ASV, and right/left ASV commissure is performed. After mapping in both the RV and LV OTs, if no sites with excellent pace-maps or early activation (earlier than −30 msec pre-QRS[14]) are seen, the CVS is typically mapped next. Injection of cold saline into the distal CVS as well as dual site pacing are helpful to identify an intramural VA origin.[15,16] Yokokawa and colleagues[15] demonstrated in 26 patients that injection of cold (room temperature) saline (with flow rates from 2 mL/min up to 60 mL/min for 10 seconds) through the tip of an ablation catheter advanced to the distal GCV during frequent VA had high sensitivity

(90%), specificity (88%), positive and negative predictive value (82% and 93%) for identifying the presence of an intramural SOO.

Furthermore, a pace-mapping correlation coefficient of less than 0.86 with the targeted VA at the earliest endocardial mapping site, and an activation time $\leq$8 msec between the 2 earliest anatomically distinct mapped areas should suggest the presence of an intramural origin[15] (AUC for both 0.85).

The earliest sites from all chambers are compared with determine the true SOO. Activation mapping of VAs with intramural sites of origin will show that the earliest endocardial sites will be relatively late, and often times there will be multiple sites from different chambers showing similar activation time. In these cases, activation mapping of the tissue between the earliest sites (ie, via CVS branches) is performed before ablation in order to try to identify the true SOO.

Mapping of the Coronary Venous System Branches

Although some operators empirically map the CVS before ablation in all patients with OT VAs,[17] it is our usual practice to proceed with mapping the CVS mainly in patients in whom no early targets are seen from the RV and LV endocardium, or in those in whom VA cannot be adequately suppressed despite ablation of early targets from the RVOT, left ventricular outflow tract (LVOT), and ASV region, mainly to minimize procedure duration as well as costs of additional catheters and sheaths required for CVS mapping because it may not be necessary in all cases.

When the decision is made to map the CVS and its branches, we typically do so via a femoral venous approach.[4] The os of the coronary sinus (CS) can be cannulated using the ablation catheter, over which a fixed-curve long sheath (SR-0) is advanced into the CS body. Alternatively, the CS can be cannulated using a J-tipped wire directly through a steerable sheath. Balloon occlusive venography (with full contrast) is then performed to visualize the CVS anatomy and identify branches of the GCV and AIV. A preprocedural CTA is also helpful to identify the course and size of the CVS branches for targeted intraprocedural mapping and catheter placement. Due to the small diameter of the distal CVS and often acute takeoff angle of its branches, the ablation catheter often cannot be advanced into the proximal septal branches. In these cases, smaller diameter multielectrode catheters (EP Star, Baylis Medical, Toronto, CA; or Map-iT; Access Point Technologies EP; Rogers, MN) or wires (Vision Wire, Biotronik;

Berlin, Germany) can be used instead to map these branches. The use of 4 to 5 French angled-tip vein selectors (Glidecath; Terumo, Shibuya, Tokyo, Japan, or Worley Vein Selector; Merit Medical, South Jordan, UT) can be helpful to select target branches to map. The location of these catheters and wires can be integrated onto the electroanatomical maps to facilitate ablation guided by anatomic proximity from opposite chambers in patients in whom the earliest SOO is localized to the proximal septal vein where the ablation catheter is unable to be advanced to the SOO in the CVS.

Nomenclature of the CVS veins and their tributaries is not uniform and different names have been assigned in the literature to veins reaching into the intramural septum. Von Lüdinghaus described in a series of autopsies a proximal septal vein that follows the first septal perforator artery. This vein was present in 55% of autopsies.[18] Our observations concur with those from von Lüdinghaus in that in the presence of a proximal septal vein, mapping of the intramural septum can be performed and identification of the SOO is facilitated; in the absence of such a vein, often the SOO of an intramural VA cannot be identified. Other terminologies have been used for these veins making comparisons of prior studies challenging. Komatsu and colleagues[19] described a series of 31 patients with OT VAs of whom the earliest SOO (with mean activation time of −34.1 ms pre-QRS) was mapped to a vein in the LV summit region (described as a communicating vein between aortic and pulmonic valves; it is unclear whether indeed this is a vein that reaches into the intramural aspect of the septum or is epicardially located) in 14 patients. Ablation using an anatomic approach from adjacent chambers guided by proximity resulted in successful elimination of VA in 10 (71%) patients. Of note, they found that the difference in activation intervals at the adjacent ablation sites compared with the earliest site in the summit communicating vein was significantly shorter in those in whom ablation was successful compared versus those in whom ablation based on anatomic proximity failed (7.6 vs 17.3 ms). Liao and colleagues[20] described 78 patients with OT VAs undergoing catheter ablation and found that 26% of these patients had VA with left bundle branch block pattern with abrupt transition in lead V3 (defined as sudden precordial transition in V3 with R-wave amplitude in V3 being more than 3 times greater than that in V2). They found this electrocardiographic pattern to be strongly predictive that the VA SOO was from the septal aspect of the LV summit, which could be targeted with ablation from the interleaflet triangle just beneath the right/left ASV junction. Kapa and colleagues,[21] reported a series of 51 patients with OT VAs of varying morphologies in whom ablation was successful from just beneath the left ASV, including nearly 40% of whom the earliest activation was from a different site and propose that VAs with SOO beneath the left ASV may have multiple exits due to heterogenous myocardial fiber orientation, resulting in different QRS morphologies. It is unclear whether the VAs described by Liao and Kapa and colleagues were indeed intramural in origin.

Ablation from Within the coronary venous system

Ablation from within the CVS can be difficult due to rapid increases in impedance during energy delivery, and in many cases, impedance cutoffs must be adjusted to permit ablation. Ablation lesions delivered from within the CVS branches have been shown to be smaller than those delivered from the endocardial RVOT or LVOT as evidenced by smaller amount of detectable late gadolinium enhancement soon on cardiac MRI 3 months post-ablation.[22] Because power is often limited by rapid impedance increases during ablation in the CVS, we have anecdotally found that the use of half normal saline as the catheter irrigant when ablating from the CVS can be helpful to create larger lesions with limited power titration. When ablating from the CVS, we typically start with low power (10–15W) and uptitrate power slowly to achieve impedance drop greater than 10 Ω.

Although the anatomy of the coronary arteries from the CTA which are integrated onto the electroanatomic map using special software such as Multi-modality Platform for Specific Imaging in Cardiology (MUSIC) can be helpful to provide a general gestalt of the course of the coronary arteries, coronary angiography should also always be considered before ablation within the CVS. A distance greater than 5 mm between the tip of the ablation catheter to the epicardial coronary arteries (in at least one fluoroscopic view) should be confirmed before ablation. In cases where the ablation catheter tip is too close to epicardial coronary arteries to safely perform radiofrequency ablation, cryoablation (−80 C° for 4–8 minutes) can be considered from the CVS because it may be less likely to result in coronary arterial injury.[23]

Fig. 1 shows an example of a patient with an intramural VA, which was successfully targeted with ablation from the proximal septal vein.[14]

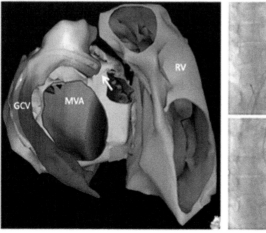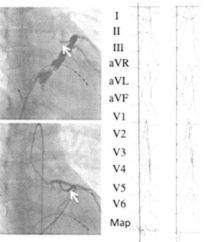

Fig. 1. Intramural PVC where ablation was delivered from within a perforator vein close to the SOO. Left panel: 3-D reconstruction of echocardiographic contours obtained by intracardiac echocardiography. Shown is a posterior view of the right ventricle (RV), the left ventricle with the mitral valve annulus (MVA) and the great cardiac vein (GCV). The ablation catheter is located in a perforator vein (*white arrow*). Middle panel: top image: Occlusive balloon venogram of the great cardiac vein. An arrow indicates the location of a proximal perforator vein draining the interventricular septum. Bottom image: Coronary angiogram of the left coronary arteries with the ablation catheter located in the perforator vein (*white arrow*). The catheter is located 5 mm below the left anterior descending artery. Right panel showing the morphology of the targeted PVC with recordings at the SOO preceding the QRS complex by 35 msec. There is a pace-map that closely matches with the spontaneous PVC morphology. Ablation at this site eliminated the patient's PVCs. (*From* Ghannam M, Liang J, Sharaf-Dabbagh G, et al. Mapping and Ablation of Intramural Ventricular Arrhythmias: A Stepwise Approach Focused on the Site of Origin. *JACC Clinical electrophysiology.* 2020;6:1339–1348, with permission.)

Strategies for Indirectly Targeting Sites that are Earliest in the coronary venous system

Not infrequently, the earliest activation site of focal OT VA is localized from within the CVS branches but ablation cannot be performed from the earliest site directly due to the inability to advance the ablation catheter to the earliest site in the CVS, inability to deliver enough power at the SOO, or proximity to epicardial coronary arteries. In these situations, alternative ablation strategies have been proposed.

One such strategy is to target the earliest breakout sites with ablation from multiple chambers. Di Biase and colleagues[24] reported a multicenter series where a strategy of sequential ablation of all early sites in multiple chambers was performed in 15 patients with intramural OT VA, with successful arrhythmia suppression in 14 (93%).

Another strategy is to map to find the true SOO by mapping the CVS branches to guide ablation based on anatomic proximity, which has been our general approach. In our experience, prioritizing identification of the SOO of intramural VAs (when feasible) is superior to ablation targeting breakout sites alone. We previously attempted to identify the SOO in 83 patients with intramural VA by mapping from within the CVS, including the perforator veins draining the intramural myocardium.[14] Occlusive CS venography was performed to delineate the anatomy of the CS branches, and an ablation catheter, multipolar mapping catheter, or a mapping wire was advanced to the target CVS branches. The actual SOO was identified in 19 (23%) of these patients with intramural focal VAs, and the VA were successfully eliminated in all 19 (100%) of these patients. In the remaining 64 patients, the SOO could not be reached for various reasons, and ablation in these patients was performed targeting the earliest breakout sites, resulting in lower success rate (67%). Of note, the SOO was significantly further away from the endocardial breakout sites than the closest anatomic sites and was actually located in another chamber than the

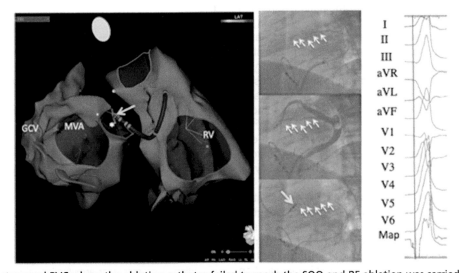

Fig. 2. Intramural PVC where the ablation catheter failed to reach the SOO and RF ablation was carried out at a site located close to the SOO in the LVOT. Left panel: 3-D reconstruction of echocardiographic contours obtained by intracardiac echocardiography. Shown is a posterior view of the right ventricle (RV), the left ventricle with the mitral valve annulus (MVA) and the great cardiac vein (GCV). The great cardiac vein and its continuation the anterior interventricular veins are colored in pink, the perforator vein is colored in lavender. The ablation catheter is located in the LVOT (yellow *arrow*). A mapping wire (gray icon) is located in the distal perforator vein (*asterisk*). Middle panel: top image: left anterior oblique (LAO) view showing selective cannulation of a perforator vein with a unipolar mapping wire (series of *white arrows*). Middle image: LAO view of an occlusive venogram showing the GCV, the AIV, and a perforator vein (series of *white arrows*). Bottom image: LAO view with the mapping wire located in the proximal perforator vein (series of *white arrows*). The ablation catheter (yellow *arrow*) is placed in the LVOT in close proximity to the tip of the mapping wire that is indicating the location of the SOO. Right panel: Recording from the mapping wire, which precedes the onset of the PVC–QRS complex by 40 msec. Radiofrequency energy was successful when ablation was performed from the ablation catheter located in the LVOT (yellow *arrow*). (*From* Ghannam M, Liang J, Sharaf-Dabbagh G, et al. Mapping and Ablation of Intramural Ventricular Arrhythmias: A Stepwise Approach Focused on the Site of Origin. *JACC Clinical electrophysiology.* 2020;6:1339–1348, with permission.)

site anatomically closest to the SOO in most patients explaining the lower success rate if the breakout sites only are targeted. Moreover, activation at the anatomically closest site to the SOO was later than at the endocardial breakout site, likely due to preferential conduction.

Fig. 2 shows an example of a patient with an intramural VA, which successfully targeted with ablation from the LVOT guided by anatomic proximity to the earliest site measured from the CVS.[14]

ADJUNCTIVE TREATMENT STRATEGIES TO TARGET INTRAMURAL ARRHYTHMIAS

Targeting of intramural VAs can be difficult due to deep intramyocardial location of the true SOO. In these cases, strategies to increase lesion size such as use of half-normal saline, delivery of longer (3–5 minute) lesions, baseline impedance modulation, and simultaneous unipolar or bipolar catheter ablation can be considered.[25–31] These strategies to increase radiofrequency energy delivery to the tissue and increase lesion size be used either in alone or in combination with each other to target intramural substrate, either targeting earliest breakout sites or the true SOO via an anatomic approach. Furthermore, alternative strategies for patients with intramural VA refractory to standard radiofrequency ablation such as infusion needle ablation, coronary venous, or arterial ethanol ablation[32,33] or noninvasive stereotactic body radiation therapy have also been used.[32–35] Surgical strategies including endoscopic robotic epicardial ablation and direct intramyocardial ethanol injection have been used successfully as well for refractory cases.[36–38]

It is important to remember that all of these strategies have not been studied in large prospective studies and may be associated with increased procedural risks, thus should only be performed carefully by experienced operators and in situations where the potential benefit of VA elimination clearly outweighs the added risk. Additional larger prospective studies are necessary to confirm the safety of these strategies.

SUMMARY

Intramural OT VAs represent a subset of VAs that can be difficult to eliminate with catheter ablation for several reasons. CMR is important to rule out scar and occult structural heart disease. In cases where activation mapping does not reveal any early sites from within the RVOT, LVOT, and ASV regions, the CVS branches should also be mapped. Although targeting of earliest breakout sites

can be effective, ideally the true SOO should be identified to facilitate direct ablation or ablation guided by anatomic proximity. Preprocedural CTA can be helpful to delineate the cardiac anatomy including the anatomy of the CVS branches and proximity to presumed VA SOO. Adjunctive strategies such as the use of half-normal saline, or simultaneous unipolar or bipolar ablation may be considered to deliver larger lesions in patients with intramural OT VAs refractory to conventional ablation strategies.

CLINICS CARE POINTS

- Intramural OT VAs can be challenging to eliminate with catheter ablation
- CMR can help to exclude occult scar and non-ischemic cardiomyopathy in patients with intramural OT VAs
- Identification of the true site of origin can facilitate successful ablation of intramural VAs

DISCLOSURE

The authors report no relevant disclosures.

REFERENCES

1. Latchamsetty R, Yokokawa M, Morady F, et al. Multicenter outcomes for catheter ablation of idiopathic premature ventricular complexes. JACC Clin Electrophysiol 2015;1:116–23.
2. Hayashi T, Liang JJ, Shirai Y, et al. Trends in successful ablation sites and outcomes of ablation for idiopathic outflow tract ventricular arrhythmias. JACC Clin Electrophysiol 2020;6:221–30.
3. Yokokawa M, Good E, Chugh A, et al. Intramural idiopathic ventricular arrhythmias originating in the intraventricular septum: mapping and ablation. Circ Arrhythm Electrophysiol 2012;5:258–63.
4. Liang JJ, Bogun F. Coronary venous mapping and catheter ablation for ventricular arrhythmias. Methodist Debakey Cardiovasc J 2021;17:13–8.
5. Bogun FM, Desjardins B, Good E, et al. Delayed-enhanced magnetic resonance imaging in nonischemic cardiomyopathy: utility for identifying the ventricular arrhythmia substrate. J Am Coll Cardiol 2009;53:1138–45.
6. Ghannam M, Siontis KC, Kim MH, et al. Risk stratification in patients with frequent premature ventricular complexes in the absence of known heart disease. Heart rhythm 2020;17:423–30.

7. Muser D, Nucifora G, Muser D, et al. Prognostic value of nonischemic ringlike left ventricular scar in patients with apparently idiopathic nonsustained ventricular arrhythmias. Circulation 2021;143: 1359–73.

8. Ghannam M, Liang JJ, Dabbagh GS, et al. Impact of intramural scar on mapping and ablation of premature ventricular complexes. JACC Clin Electrophysiol 2021;7:733–41.

9. Ghannam M, Liang JJ, Attili A, et al. Cardiac magnetic resonance imaging and ventricular tachycardias involving the sinuses of valsalva in patients with nonischemic cardiomyopathy. JACC Clin Electrophysiol 2021;7:1243–53.

10. Liang JJ, D'Souza BA, Betensky BP, et al. Importance of the interventricular septum as part of the ventricular tachycardia substrate in nonischemic cardiomyopathy. JACC Clin Electrophysiol 2018;4: 1155–62.

11. Ibrahim EH, Runge M, Stojanovska J, et al. Optimized cardiac magnetic resonance imaging inversion recovery sequence for metal artifact reduction and accurate myocardial scar assessment in patients with cardiac implantable electronic devices. World J Radiol 2018;10:100–7.

12. Briceño DF, Enriquez A, Liang JJ, et al. Septal coronary venous mapping to guide substrate characterization and ablation of intramural septal ventricular arrhythmia. JACC Clin Electrophysiol 2019;5: 789–800.

13. Ghannam M, Siontis KC, Kim HM, et al. Factors predictive for delayed enhancement in cardiac resonance imaging in patients undergoing catheter ablation of premature ventricular complexes. Heart Rhythm O2 2021;2:64–72.

14. Ghannam M, Liang J, Sharaf-Dabbagh G, et al. Mapping and ablation of intramural ventricular arrhythmias: a stepwise approach focused on the site of origin. JACC Clin Electrophysiol 2020;6: 1339–48.

15. Yokokawa M, Morady F, Bogun F. Injection of cold saline for diagnosis of intramural ventricular arrhythmias. Heart Rhythm 2016;13:78–82.

16. Yokokawa M, Yon Jung D, Hero AO III, et al. Single- and dual-site pace mapping of idiopathic septal intramural ventricular arrhythmias. Heart Rhythm 2016;13(1):72–7.

17. Pothineni NVK, Garg L, Guandalini G, et al. A novel approach to mapping and ablation of septal outflow tract ventricular arrhythmias: insights from multipolar intraseptal recordings. Heart Rhythm 2021;18: 1445–51.

18. von Ludinghausen M. The venous drainage of the human myocardium. Adv Anat Embryol Cell Biol 2003;168(I-VIII):1–104.

19. Komatsu Y, Nogami A, Shinoda Y, et al. Idiopathic ventricular arrhythmias originating from the vicinity of the communicating vein of cardiac venous systems at the left ventricular summit. Circ Arrhythm Electrophysiol 2018;11:e005386.

20. Liao H, Wei W, Tanager KS, et al. Left ventricular summit arrhythmias with an abrupt V(3) transition: anatomy of the aortic interleaflet triangle vantage point. Heart rhythm 2021;18:10–9.

21. Kapa S, Mehra N, Deshmukh AJ, et al. Left sinus of valsalva-electroanatomic basis and outcomes with ablation for outflow tract arrhythmias. J Cardiovasc Electrophysiol 2020;31:952–9.

22. Candemir B, Ozyurek E, Vurgun K, et al. Effect of radiofrequency on epicardial myocardium after ablation of ventricular arrhythmias from within coronary sinus. Pacing Clin Electrophysiol 2018;41:1060–8.

23. Nagashima K, Choi EK, Lin KY, et al. Ventricular arrhythmias near the distal great cardiac vein: challenging arrhythmia for ablation. Circ Arrhythmia Electrophysiol 2014;7:906–12.

24. Di Biase L, Romero J, Zado ES, et al. Variant of ventricular outflow tract ventricular arrhythmias requiring ablation from multiple sites: intramural origin. Heart Rhythm 2019;16:724–32.

25. Nguyen DT, Gerstenfeld EP, Tzou WS, et al. Radiofrequency ablation using an open irrigated electrode cooled with half-normal saline. JACC Clin Electrophysiol 2017;3:1103–10.

26. Nguyen DT, Tzou WS, Sandhu A, et al. Prospective multicenter experience with cooled radiofrequency ablation using high impedance irrigant to target deep myocardial substrate refractory to standard ablation. JACC Clin Electrophysiol 2018;4:1176–85.

27. Liang JJ, Santangeli P, Marchlinski FE. Radiofrequency ablation in dense ventricular scar-Longer continuous lesions may be beneficial. J Cardiovasc Electrophysiol 2020;31:1891.

28. Shapira-Daniels A, Barkagan M, Rottmann M, et al. Modulating the baseline impedance: an adjunctive technique for maximizing radiofrequency lesion dimensions in deep and intramural ventricular substrate: an adjunctive technique for maximizing radiofrequency lesion dimensions in deep and intramural ventricular substrate. Circ Arrhythmia Electrophysiol 2019;12:e007336.

29. Yang J, Liang J, Shirai Y, et al. Outcomes of simultaneous unipolar radiofrequency catheter ablation for intramural septal ventricular tachycardia in nonischemic cardiomyopathy. Heart Rhythm 2019;16: 863–70.

30. Igarashi M, Nogami A, Fukamizu S, et al. Acute and long-term results of bipolar radiofrequency catheter ablation of refractory ventricular arrhythmias of deep intramural origin. Heart Rhythm 2020;17: 1500–7.

31. Futyma P, Santangeli P, Pürerfellner H, et al. Anatomic approach with bipolar ablation between the left pulmonic cusp and left ventricular outflow

tract for left ventricular summit arrhythmias. Heart Rhythm 2020;17:1519–27.

32. Tokuda M, Sobieszczyk P, Eisenhauer AC, et al. Transcoronary ethanol ablation for recurrent ventricular tachycardia after failed catheter ablation: an update. Circ Arrhythm Electrophysiol 2011;4: 889–96.

33. Kreidieh B, Rodríguez-Mañero M, Schurmann P, et al. Retrograde coronary venous ethanol infusion for ablation of refractory ventricular tachycardia. Circ Arrhythmia Electrophysiol 2016;9. https://doi.org/10.1161/CIRCEP.116.004352.

34. Stevenson WG, Tedrow UB, Reddy V, et al. Infusion needle radiofrequency ablation for treatment of refractory ventricular arrhythmias. J Am Coll Cardiol 2019;73:1413–25.

35. Cuculich PS, Schill MR, Kashani R, et al. Noninvasive cardiac radiation for ablation of ventricular tachycardia. N Engl J Med 2017;377:2325–36.

36. Aziz Z, Moss JD, Jabbarzadeh M, et al. Totally endoscopic robotic epicardial ablation of refractory left ventricular summit arrhythmia: first-in-man. Heart Rhythm 2017;14:135–8.

37. Kowlgi GN, Arghami A, Crestanello JA, et al. Direct intramyocardial ethanol injection for premature ventricular contraction arising from the inaccessible left ventricular summit. JACC Clin Electrophysiol 2021;7(12):1647–8.

38. Yang G, Shao Y, Gu W, et al. Surgical ablation supplemented by ethanol injection for ventricular tachycardia refractory to percutaneous ablation. J Cardiovasc Electrophysiol 2021;32:2462–70.

Bipolar Radiofrequency Catheter Ablation of Left Ventricular Summit Arrhythmias

Piotr Futyma, MD, PhD[a],*, William H. Sauer, MD[b]

KEYWORDS

- Left ventricular summit • Bipolar ablation • Ventricular tachycardia • Premature ventricular complex

KEY POINTS

- Left ventricular (LV) summit architecture may prevent sufficient heating of the targeted area during standard radiofrequency catheter ablation.
- Bipolar ablation can overcome some problems of ablation of LV summit arrhythmias and increase a chance of achieving a transmural lesion.
- Targeting the LV summit area using bipolar ablation provides several configurations.

BACKGROUND

The left ventricular (LV) summit is a frequent source of origin of ventricular arrhythmias (VA), and thus a common target for radiofrequency catheter ablation (RFCA). Challenging anatomic and morphologic conditions of the LV summit architecture and its surrounding sites, including proximity of major coronary arteries, presence of substantial epicardial fat layer, and fibrotic components of the aortic and pulmonic valves, may prevent sufficient heating of the targeted LV ostium area using standard RFCA approach.[1] Radiofrequency (RF) applications applied near the LV summit can be performed from accessible adjacent structures, such as subvalvular left ventricular outflow tract (LVOT), great cardiac vein (GCV), anterior interventricular veins (AIV), or aortic and pulmonic cusps. Nevertheless, long-term efficacy of RFCA drops substantially if a multisite ablation for such LV summit VA is required.[2] Alternatively, RF current can be delivered in bipolar fashion, between distal electrodes of 2 separate ablation catheters (AC), as this will result in higher

RF current delivery in the area of interest. Bipolar ablation can result in higher likelihood of efficacy for ablation of LV summit arrhythmias from inaccessible regions and lesion transmurally. In this review, the authors describe the present approaches for bipolar radiofrequency catheter ablation (Bi-RFCA) of the LV summit VAs refractory to standard approaches.

From a historical standpoint, bipolar ablation in the very early era of RFCA was initially used for treatment of lateral accessory pathways, as an alternative for direct current ablation.[3] In this approach, one of the solid-tip electrodes was advanced into the coronary sinus (CS), and the second one was positioned in the opposing endocardial mitral annulus. This approach was abandoned because of poor blood flow in the CS, causing overheating and impedance mismatch resulting in nonuniform lesion creation. Thus, most accessory pathway ablation cases from the study by Jackman and colleagues[3] were completed using the standard unipolar approach. However, Bi-RFCA has subsequently been described for the treatment of refractory

Conflict of interest: none.
[a] Medical College, University of Rzeszów and St. Joseph's Heart Rhythm Center, Anny Jagiellonki 17, Rzeszów 35-623, Poland; [b] Cardiac Arrhythmia Service, Brigham and Women's Hospital, 75 Francis Street, Boston, MA 02115, USA
* Corresponding author.
E-mail address: piotr.futyma@gmail.com

Card Electrophysiol Clin 15 (2023) 57–62
https://doi.org/10.1016/j.ccep.2022.07.001
1877-9182/23/© 2022 The Author(s). Published by Elsevier Inc. This is an open access article under the CC BY-NC-ND license (http://creativecommons.org/licenses/by-nc-nd/4.0/).

posteroseptal accessory pathways.[4] In addition, Bi-RFCA has also been used for ablation of aortic cusps and septal and free wall VTs[5,6] and most recently for septal outflow tract and LV summit arrhythmias.[7–9]

Biophysical rationale for bipolar ablation of LV summit VA comes from complex anatomic relations in the LV ostium area, which contribute to impaired RFCA efficacy. One study showed that the epicardial fat layer can reach up to 12.1 mm, and this can prevent conventional RF delivery to effectively treat an underlying LV summit arrhythmia.[10] The presence of the epicardial adipose tissue illustrates the need for improved RF energy delivery, which has been demonstrated in ex vivo studies.[11] Alternatively, Bi-RFCA can lead to increased lesion depth in cases of moderate levels of adipose tissue.[12,13] In addition, the presence of multiple sites surrounding LV summit, which are accessible to classic ablation approaches, provides a broad spectrum of configurations for Bi-RFCA, leaving the field clear for numerous approaches.

ANATOMIC ASPECTS OF THE LEFT VENTRICULAR SUMMIT AND VARIABILITY OF BIPOLAR ABLATION CONFIGURATIONS

From the anatomic standpoint, Bi-RFCA targeting the LV summit area provides several configurations (**Fig. 1**). Locations capable of hosting 1 of 2 ACs for Bi-RFCA include the following:

- Aortic cusps
- Left/right interleaflet triangle of the aortic valve
- Left ventricular outflow tract (LVOT)
- Right ventricular outflow tract (RVOT)
- Left pulmonic cusp (LPC)
- Great cardiac vein (GCV)
- Anterior intraventricular vein (AIV)

Table 1 summarizes to-date literature reporting outcomes of Bi-RFCA at the LV summit area. Although multiple sites suitable for bipolar ablation introduces opportunities for RF delivery through the LV summit, several challenges should be taken into account. In one of the initial reports, Bi-RFCA was performed between the left aortic cusp and subvalvular LVOT.[5] Such an approach requires double arterial access for both AC, leaving no space for additional arterial access necessary for performing a coronary angiogram at the time of ablation, which is often necessary for exact determination of coronary artery route, in order to avoid its injury. Distance above 5 mm from the tip of each AC to coronaries in 2 projections and avoiding the presence of coronary artery in between the 2 catheters used for Bi-RFCA should be provided.

As the aortic root and subvalvular region of the LVOT are delineated by only thin leaflets of the aortic valve, it should be also taken into account that the intercatheter distance during Bi-RFCA can be too close, and this may result in thrombus formation or RF current preferential conduction through blood. For similar reasons, Bi-RFCA at the intercatheter distance less than 5 mm was avoided in 1 study.[14]

BIPOLAR ABLATION OF THE SEPTAL REGION OF THE LEFT VENTRICULAR SUMMIT

Anteromedial LV summit VAs will include the common target of the upper interventricular septum, also called the septal portion. In one of earliest studies on Bi-RFCA, such an approach was performed successfully in 4 patients without complications and with a notable success rate of 75%.[7] Despite the fact that the investigators use the nomenclature of "outflow tract" PVC/VT in their study, electrocardiographic (ECG) features provided by Teh and colleagues[7] demonstrate abrupt V3 transition zone are suggestive for typical LV summit VA.[15] The possible advantage of ablation between RVOT and LVOT is the fact that it does not require any special maneuvers with AC. Second, when bipolar ablation between RVOT and LVOT is performed, both catheters operate in a similar blood pool, making the impedance mismatch affect less impactful on lesion creation, thus allowing unconstrained energy and RF time titration. However, such an approach may not reach some VA originating in the inaccessible LV summit area covered by the left anterior descending artery (LAD) of the left main coronary artery or septal perforators. The most lateral part of the LV summit appears also to be out of range of Bi-RFCA RVOT-LVOT catheter configuration. The use of large-tip electrodes can provide some advantages when targeting anteromedial LV summit; however, literature data on utilization of two 8-mm catheters are scarce.[16]

BIPOLAR ABLATION OF THE LEFT VENTRICULAR SUMMIT UTILIZING CORONARY VEINS

Coronary veins, particularly GCV and AIV, are a common target for mapping and ablation of the LV summit arrhythmias. Nevertheless, as mentioned previously, classic unipolar ablation can be insufficient to achieve desired lesion depth, mainly because of 2 reasons:

- Epicardial adipose tissue
- Coronary vein caliber

A	**B**	**C**
Antero-medial LV summit	Inaccessible LV summit	Lateral LV summit

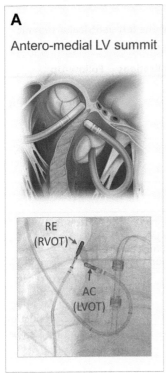
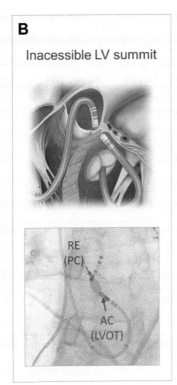
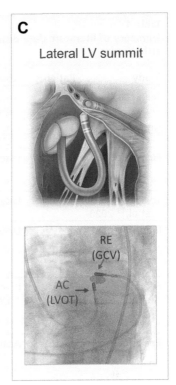

Fig. 1. Representative fluoroscopic images depicting approaches of the LV summit Bi-RFCA. (*A*) Ablation of the anteromedial LV summit. Bi-RFCA is performed between 2 AC: the first 8-mm AC is positioned using reversed U-curve in the RVOT and serves as a return electrode (RE) during Bi-RFCA, and the second, open irrigated U-curved AC is located in the subaortic region of LVOT. (*B*) Ablation of the inaccessible LV summit. Bi-RFCA is performed between 2 open-irrigated AC: the first AC (acting as RE) is positioned using reversed U-curve in the LPC and the second U-curved AC is located in the subaortic region of LVOT. PC, pulmonic cusp. (*C*) Bi-RFCA of more lateral LV summit aspect. An open irrigated U-curved AC is located in LVOT, whereas a nonirrigated 8-mm-tip AC is positioned in the GCV. This catheter serves as RE. The use of a large 8-mm tip is justified to minimize the impedance mismatch effect.

By advancing one of the AC into GCV/AIV and a second to the opposite endocardial LVOT or aortic cusp, the path of RF current can be redirected toward LVS using Bi-RFCA.[17] This Bi-RFCA configuration can result in reduction of VA burden and lesion transmurality.[8] The challenges regarding advancing an AC to a vessel of a small diameter can be overcome using a telescopic approach.[18] Issues during Bi-RFCA, such as electrode overheating in the GCV/AIV, impedance variability, or impedance increase resulting in premature Bi-RFCA application termination, can be solved by advancing an 8-mm-tip catheter into the coronary vein.[19] A possible overheating and subsequent char formation on a nonirrigated AC should be taken into account.[20,21]

BIPOLAR ABLATION OF THE INACCESSIBLE LEFT VENTRICULAR SUMMIT

RFCA of arrhythmias arising from the most superior aspect of the LV summit region, which has been defined as "inaccessible" owing to proximity to the left main coronary artery and its bifurcation into the left anterior descending and left circumflex coronary arteries together with a thick layer of epicardial fat, is particularly challenging, as direct ablation at the earliest site of activation is frequently not possible. Moreover, RF delivery from GCV/AIV would violate the 5-mm rule for safe distance from a coronary artery. Recently, a reversed U-curve technique was implemented for mapping of the pulmonic valve cusps.[22,23] This technique allows positioning of the tip of the AC anatomically below the level of the proximal LAD artery. However, the success of this approach alone for refractory LV summit PVC/VT remains anecdotal.[24] In these patients, with LV summit VAs arising from an inaccessible region and refractory to conventional RFCA, a purely anatomic approach using Bi-RFA from the LPC and opposite LVOT can be an effective alternative approach.[9] Advancing the LPC using U-curved AC can be supported by the use of a long sheath.

Table 1
Summary of literature data describing outcomes of bipolar ablation of the left ventricular summit arrhythmias

Study	Patients	Ablation Targets	Power (W)	Complications	Follow-Up
Teh et al,[7]	4	Anteromedial LV summit	Up to 35	None	75% success during follow-up
Nguyen et al,[25] 2016	1	Anteromedial LV summit	50	None	Recurrence
Futyma et al,[8]	4	Lateral LV summit	24 ± 6	None	No VT recurrence, 83% PVC burden reduction
Tokioka et al,[19] 2020	3	Lateral LV summit	35–40	None	Acute success
Igarashi et al,[26] 2020	4	LV summit	Up to 45	None in the LV summit cohort	Acute success
Futyma et al,[9] 2020	7	Inaccessible LV summit	36 ± 7	None	No VT recurrence in VT group, overall 84% PVC burden reduction
Enriquez et al,[27] 2019	1	Anteromedial LV summit	Up to 45 with half normal saline (HNS) irrigation	None	No PVC after 4 wk
Sauer et al,[29] 2018	1	Anteromedial LV summit	50	None	No VT after 6 mo

Remote magnetic navigation can be particularly useful for reversed U-curve mapping and ablation above the pulmonic valve.[25] Safety concerns should include a possible dislodgement of U-curved AC during Bi-RFCA, which can especially occur during deep breath.

In summary, for each case, the anatomic configuration of Bi-RFCA should be determined individually, based on ECG characteristics, anatomic features, cavital and sometimes intramural mapping outcomes, as well as effects of prior ablations on transient VA suppression. The combination of listed features can help to determine the most optimal Bi-RFCA approach.

COMBINATION OF BIPOLAR ABLATION WITH OTHER EMERGING TECHNIQUES

Bipolar ablation can be freely combined with other ablation methods. The most straightforward combination is additional unipolar ablation toward LV summit during the Bi-RFCA procedure, which frequently precedes other techniques tailored to the deep intramural arrhythmia sites. Other techniques include concomitant alcohol ablation.[26] Effects of Bi-RFCA can be augmented with irrigation of AC using low- or nonionic coolants, such as half normal saline (HNS)[27] or dextrose-5 in water.[9] Mapping wires or microcatheters in the septal perforators can be helpful not only for better definition of exact Bi-RFCA target but also to enhance RF delivery using the antenna effect.[28]

FUTURE DIRECTIONS

Standard unipolar RFCA remains the most common strategy for ablative treatment of LV summit arrhythmias. However, some patients with intramural LVS PVC/VT site of origin can benefit from bipolar ablation implemented at an earlier stage of ablative treatment. Optimization of catheter shape, size, and interelectrode distance using dedicated equipment can allow for the safe delivery of Bi-RFCA of the LV summit VA earlier.

LIMITATIONS

A few limitations are worth highlighting. First, the clinical data of LV summit Bi-RFCA come from small retrospective multicenter studies. Second, the long-term efficacy of LV summit Bi-RFCA remains unknown. Last, outcomes of LVS Bi-RFCA can be dependent of equipment used and may differ between centers. Bi-RFCA often involves the off-label use of equipment designed for standard unipolar ablation, limiting the utility of this approach in some centers.

CLINICS CARE POINTS

- Locations capable of hosting 1 of 2 ablation catheters during bipolar ablation of the left ventricular summit include aortic and pulmonic cusps, interleaflet triangle, left and right ventricular outflow tract, and coronary veins.
- The use of large-tip electrodes can be especially useful when coronary veins are involved during bipolar ablation.
- Particular attention should be given to the presence of the nearby coronary arteries during bipolar ablation of the left ventricular summit arrhythmias.

REFERENCES

1. Yamada T, McElderry HT, Doppalapudi H, et al. Idiopathic ventricular arrhythmias originating from the left ventricular summit: anatomic concepts relevant to ablation. Circ Arrhythm Electrophysiol 2010;3(6): 616–23.
2. Chung FP, Lin CY, Shirai Y, et al. Outcomes of catheter ablation of ventricular arrhythmia originating from the left ventricular summit: a multicenter study. Heart Rhythm 2020;17(7):1077–83.
3. Jackman WM, Wang XZ, Friday KJ, et al. Catheter ablation of accessory atrioventricular pathways (Wolff-Parkinson-White syndrome) by radiofrequency current. N Engl J Med 1991;324(23): 1605–11.
4. Bashir Y, Heald SC, O'Nunain S, et al. Radiofrequency current delivery by way of a bipolar tricuspid annulus-mitral annulus electrode configuration for ablation of posteroseptal accessory pathways. J Am Coll Cardiol 1993;22:550–6.
5. Merino JL, Peinado R, Ramirez L, et al. Ablation of idiopathic ventricular tachycardia by bipolar radiofrequency current application between the left aortic sinus and the left ventricle. Europace 2000;2(4): 350–4.
6. Koruth JS, Dukkipati S, Miller MA, et al. Bipolar irrigated radiofrequency ablation: a therapeutic option for refractory intramural atrial and ventricular tachycardia circuits. Heart Rhythm 2012;9(12):1932–41.
7. Teh AW, Reddy VY, Koruth JS, et al. Bipolar radiofrequency catheter ablation for refractory ventricular outflow tract arrhythmias. J Cardiovasc Electrophysiol 2014;25(10):1093–9.
8. Futyma P, Sander J, Ciąpała K, et al. Bipolar radiofrequency ablation delivered from coronary veins and adjacent endocardium for treatment of refractory left ventricular summit arrhythmias. J Interv Card Electrophysiol 2020;58(3):307–13.
9. Futyma P, Santangeli P, Pürerfellner H, et al. Anatomic approach with bipolar ablation between the left pulmonic cusp and left ventricular outflow tract for left ventricular summit arrhythmias. Heart Rhythm 2020;17(9):1519–27.
10. Candemir B, Ozyurek E, Vurgun K, et al. Effect of radiofrequency on epicardial myocardium after ablation of ventricular arrhythmias from within coronary sinus. Pacing Clin Electrophysiol 2018;41: 1060–8.
11. d'Avila A, Houghtaling C, Gutierrez P, et al. Catheter ablation of ventricular epicardial tissue: a comparison of standard and cooled-tip radiofrequency energy. Circulation 2004;109(19):2363–9.
12. Zipse MM, Edward JA, Zheng L, et al. Impact of epicardial adipose tissue and catheter ablation strategy on biophysical parameters and ablation lesion characteristics. J Cardiovasc Electrophysiol 2020;31(5):1114–24.
13. Hong KN, Russo MJ, Liberman EA, et al. Effect of epicardial fat on ablation performance: a three-energy source comparison. J Card Surg 2007; 22(6):521–4.
14. Della Bella P, Peretto G, Paglino G, et al. Bipolar radiofrequency ablation for ventricular tachycardias originating from the interventricular septum: Safety and efficacy in a pilot cohort study. Heart Rhythm 2020;17(12):2111–8.
15. Liao H, Wei W, Tanager KS, et al. Left ventricular summit arrhythmias with an abrupt V3 transition: Anatomy of the aortic interleaflet triangle vantage point. Heart Rhythm 2021;18(1):10–9.
16. Ferraz AP, Andere TE, Gonçalves ALM, et al. Bipolar radiofrequency ablation of septal ventricular tachycardia in a patient with dilated cardiomyopathy using two 8-mm tip catheters-case report. J Interv Card Electrophysiol 2022;9. https://doi.org/10.1007/s10840-022-01150-y.
17. Futyma P, Wysokińska A, Sander J, et al. Bipolar Endo-epicardial radiofrequency ablation of arrhythmia originating from the left ventricular summit. Circ J 2018;82(6):1721–2.
18. Baszko A, Kałmucki P, Siminiak T, et al. Telescopic coronary sinus cannulation for mapping and ethanol ablation of arrhythmia originating from left ventricular summit. Cardiol J 2020;27(3):312–5.
19. Tokioka S, Fukamizu S, Kawamura I, et al. Bipolar radiofrequency catheter ablation between the left

ventricular endocardium and great cardiac vein for refractory ventricular premature complexes originating from the left ventricular summit. J Arrhythm 2020;36(2):363–6.

20. Futyma P, Głuszczyk R, Futyma M, et al. Right atrial position of a return electrode for bipolar ablation of the left posterosuperior process ventricular tachycardia. Pacing Clin Electrophysiol 2019;42(4):474–7.

21. Futyma P, Ciąpała K, Głuszczyk R, et al. Bipolar ablation of refractory atrial and ventricular arrhythmias: Importance of temperature values of intracardiac return electrodes. J Cardiovasc Electrophysiol 2019;30(9):1718–26.

22. Heeger CH, Kuck KH, Ouyang F. Catheter ablation of pulmonary sinus cusp-derived ventricular arrhythmias by the reversed U-curve technique. J Cardiovasc Electrophysiol 2017;28(7):776–7.

23. Zhang J, Tang C, Zhang Y, et al. Pulmonary sinus cusp mapping and ablation: a new concept and approach for idiopathic right ventricular outflow tract arrhythmias. Heart Rhythm 2018;15:38–45.

24. Futyma P, Moroka K, Derndorfer M, et al. Left pulmonary cusp ablation of refractory ventricular arrhythmia originating from the inaccessible summit. Europace 2019;21(8):1253.

25. Nguyen DT, Tzou WS, Brunnquell M, et al. Clinical and biophysical evaluation of variable bipolar configurations during radiofrequency ablation for treatment of ventricular arrhythmias. Heart Rhythm 2016;13(11):2161–71.

26. Igarashi M, Nogami A, Fukamizu S, et al. Acute and long-term results of bipolar radiofrequency catheter ablation of refractory ventricular arrhythmias of deep intramural origin. Heart Rhythm 2020;17(9):1500–7.

27. Enriquez A, Neira V, Bakker D, et al. Bipolar ablation with half normal saline for deep intramural outflow tract premature ventricular contraction. Heartrhythm Case Rep 2019;5(8):436–9.

28. Waight MC, Wiles BM, Li AC, et al. Bipolar radiofrequency ablation of septal ventricular tachycardia facilitated by an intramural catheter. JACC Case Rep 2021;3(8):1119–24.

29. Sauer PJ, Kunkel MJ, Nguyen DT, et al. Successful ablation of ventricular tachycardia arising from a midmyocardial septal outflow tract site utilizing a simplified bipolar ablation setup. Heartrhythm Case Rep 2018;5(2):105–8.

Retrograde Coronary Venous Ethanol Infusion for Ablation of Refractory Left Ventricular Summit Arrhythmias

Thomas Flautt, DO, Miguel Valderrábano, MD, PhD*

KEYWORDS

- Alcohol • Ablation • Annular vein

KEY POINTS

- Coronary veins can be used to reach substrates of ventricular arrhythmias.
- Venous ethanol ablation of focal ventricular arrhythmias from the left ventricular summit requires detailed understanding of the individual anatomy.
- Double-balloon approaches can be useful for large substrate ablation.

WHY ETHANOL?

Ethanol (CH_3CH_2OH) is a short-chain alcohol, water-soluble compound that rapidly crosses the cell membranes. When cells are exposed to high concentrations, ethanol solubilizes the cell membranes and alters the tertiary protein structures, leading to immediate cell destruction.[1,2] Most of the fluid membranes, including those that are low in cholesterol, are the most easily solubilized by ethanol. Ethanol interferes with the packing of molecules in the phospholipid bilayer of the cell membrane, thus increasing membrane fluidity. Additional subcellular effects have been reported, including biochemical alterations of mitochondria such as decreases in mitochondrial adenosine triophosphate (ATPase) activity, [3] leading to mitochondrial dysfunction, as reported in ethanol-induced cardiomyopathy,[4] and it may not be significant in the acute setting.[5]

Intravascular ethanol infusion may have additional effects related to vascular damage with sclerosis of the injected vessel, which follows routinely after infusion. In intra-arterial infusions, tissue ischemia and infarction of the injected territory are expected to play a role in ethanol's therapeutic effect.[6] Venous sclerosis is also to be expected.[7]

HISTORY OF CHEMICAL ABLATION FOR VENTRICULAR ARRHYTHMIAS

The first successful ventricular tachycardia ablation with ethanol was reported in dogs by Chilson and colleagues[8] and transcoronary by Inoue and colleagues[9], both in Zipes' animal laboratory. In their animal study, focal ventricular tachycardia induced by intramyocardial injection of aconitine was suppressed by ethanol (approximately 50% concentration) or phenol injection delivered into the artery supplying the aconitine-injected myocardial tissue. Successful ventricular tachycardia elimination was correlated with myocardial necrosis and arterial thrombus formation, which were not achieved by lower (25%) ethanol concentrations. Brugada and colleagues[10] reported effective cure of ventricular tachycardia by intracoronary arterial ethanol infusion in three patients who had remained in incessant ventricular tachycardia refraction to multiple treatment modalities. Kay and colleagues[11] prospectively evaluated the

Division of Cardiac Electrophysiology, Department of Cardiology, Houston Methodist DeBakey Heart and Vascular Center, Houston Methodist Hospital, Houston, TX, USA
* Corresponding author. 6550 Fannin Street, Suite 1801, Houston, TX 77030.
E-mail address: mvalderrabano@houstonmethodist.org

Card Electrophysiol Clin 15 (2023) 63–74
https://doi.org/10.1016/j.ccep.2022.10.003
1877-9182/23/© 2023 Elsevier Inc. All rights reserved.

clinical utility of intra-arterial ethanol infusion for ventricular tachycardia in 23 patients. They found that ventricular tachycardia could be terminated by injections of saline solution or contrast medium in 11 of the 21 patients in whom the protocol could be completed. Ethanol was infused in 10 of these patients and led to the acute elimination of ventricular tachycardia inducibility in 90% of them.[11] After repeating the electrophysiology study, inducibility recovered in two other patients, yielding an overall success of 70%. Associated complications included complete atrioventricular block in four patients (40%) and pericarditis in one patient. Initial ethanol dose and concentration ("absolute" or 96% to 98%) appeared to be arbitrarily selected. Haines and colleagues[12] performed a systematic study in dogs addressing these issues, testing different concentrations (0%, 10%, 25%, 50%, 75%, and 100%): as the ethanol concentration increased, the ablation vessels were more persistently occluded and the size of identifiable myocardial lesions is increased significantly with increasing ethanol concentration, although there was significant variability within groups.[6]

TRANSCORONARY ETHANOL ABLATION: CURRENT ROLE

Although radiofrequency catheter ablation (RFCA) with epicardial and endocardial mapping can successfully treat most refractory VTs, there remains a subset of patients whose ventricular tachycardia (VT) is not amenable to RFCA. These are mainly VTs with deep midmyocardial origin in which radiofrequency energy cannot reach with sufficient therapeutic effect. Another group is patients with epicardial circuits and a history of heart surgery, making epicardial access difficult if not impossible. In a large series of RF-refractory VTs, Kumar showed transcoronary ethanol ablation (TCEA)'s value in rescuing these otherwise impossible-to-treat patients.[13]

Although TCEA is reasonably successful in treating RCFA-refractory VTs, there are technical difficulties and potential complications inherent to coronary artery instrumentation such as coronary arterial dissection, thrombosis, and myocardial infarction. Other complications are related to the spillage of ethanol to nontargeted myocardium resulting in interventricular conduction blocks, and infarction of non-selected regions.[14,15]

RETROGRADE CORONARY VENOUS ETHANOL ABLATION

Recognizing these limitations of intra-arterial delivery, Inoue and colleagues[9] originally described that coronary sinus (CS) phenol infusion in dogs led to 'considerable' subendocardial necrosis, but there were no additional descriptions. Wright and colleagues[16] explored the retrograde venous approach in a canine model. Balloon occlusion of the distal anterior inter-ventricular vein or the distal great cardiac vein (GCV) was performed and then ethanol was infused at 1.5, 3, and 5 mL. They found that transmural lesions could be achieved when infused ethanol volumes were approximately 3 mL, and hypothesized that for smaller volumes, collateral flow via Thebesian veins into the left ventricular (LV) cavity could prevent ethanol from reaching the capillaries, where its ablative action would reach the myocardial cells.[6]

Venous Versus Arterial Ethanol

Retrograde coronary venous ethanol ablation (RCVEA) can be favored over TCEA for multiple reasons. With a venous approach, a relatively unobstructed access to the capillary bed is available even in patients with severe coronary artery disease. There is less risk associated with cannulation of the coronary veins than of the coronary arteries. There is also less risk of damaging collateral arteries. RCVEA also remains a feasible option in patients in which previous coronary artery bypass graft may limit access to the pericardium and to the coronary arteries for arterial ethanol ablation. However, there remain uncertainties regarding the safety and utility of RCVEA that this initial report cannot address. Although the size of the ventricular vein selected for ethanol infusion can be expected to correlate with the extent of tissue reached and ablated by ethanol, there is no control as to the extent of myocardial tissue ablated by ethanol, which may be excessive. In addition, the venous anatomy may not always provide access to the targeted myocardium.

The coronary venous anatomy is extremely redundant. Aside from venous return to the CS, Thebesian veins can drain directly into the LV cavity.[16] Within the epicardial venous system, collateral veins abound, communicating epicardial veins with one another and the CS (**Fig. 1**). When targeting the myocardium with ethanol, it is important to use a vein with a direct connection to capillaries to avoid ethanol shunting. Collateral veins may be present at baseline injection.

In some cases, collateral veins disappear after ethanol, whereas in others, they became more prominent. It has been hypothesized that ethanol obliterates capillaries. Collateral veins arising after the capillary territory is obliterated by ethanol will disappear after ethanol whereas those collateral veins arising before the capillaries may become

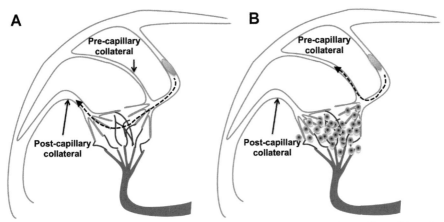

Fig. 1. (*A*) Postcapillary collateral is visible before ethanol ablation. (*B*) Postcapillary collateral is no longer visible and a precapillary collateral is visible after ethanol administration.

more prominent **Fig. 1** shows a schematic illustrating this concept.[17]

This is particularly true for VT originating from the LV summit, where an intramural origin, proximity to coronary vessels, and inaccessibility to the epicardial approach limit radiofrequency ablation (RFA) success.[18]

VENOUS ETHANOL FOR LEFT VENTRICULAR SUMMIT
Anatomy

Intramural branches of the coronary venous system offer a unique opportunity for reaching arrhythmogenic foci, and RCVEA can effectively treat ventricular arrhythmias ventricular annulars (VAs).[17,19,20] Successful ventricular ethanol ablation (VEA) requires a comprehensive appreciation of the morphologic arrangement of cardiac veins, particularly of the LV summit. The number and location of coronary tributaries vary, and their size and course are also notoriously diverse.[21] Previous studies have used computed tomography (CT) to describe the relationship between the coronary venous and arterial systems and the main tributaries of the CS[21,22]; however, the epicardial and intramural branches of left ventricular summit (LVS) tributaries have not been studied in detail. LVS vein nomenclature often is imprecise and inconsistent, as LVS veins are referred to as "communicating veins" or "septal perforators,"[23–25] without discriminating their relationship to neighboring structures such as the mitral annulus, aortic root, right ventricular (RV) outflow tract (RVOT), and LVOT.

Our group compiled occlusive venograms of 53 patients undergoing RCVEA for LVS VAs. We analyzed the angiographic anatomy of all 53 patients considered for LVS VEA and correlated

vein location with the mapped geometry of the anterior intraventricular vein (AIV), left ventricular outflow tract (LVOT), and right ventricular outflow tract (RVOT) on three-dimensional (3D) (CARTO) maps.

Below is a comprehensive review of the venous anatomy.

Great cardiac vein–anterior interventricular vein transition
The transition from the GCV to the anterior interventricular vein (AIV) is a critical aspect of the LVS venous anatomy. Angulations in the GCV–AIV transition have previously been measured.[22] We broadly dichotomize this transition in two categories: angled versus nonangled transition (**Fig. 2**). For the electrophysiologist attempting to reach the LVS area through the GCV or AIV, this is important because a steep angle at the GCV–AIV transition makes difficult cannulation with large or stiff multipolar catheters. In our experience, sharply angled GCV–AIV transitions can make cannulation with a DecaNav (Biosense Webster) catheter difficult, and advancement of a subselector left internal mammary artery (LIMA) or Judkins right 4 (JR4) into the proximal AIV can be unstable and counterproductive when trying to direct their tip toward septal branches.[26]

Left ventricular annular vein
LV annular (LVA) vein: The LVA was present in 19 of 53 venograms (36%). Defined as a branch of the GCV arising before the GCV–AIV junction, in the mitral annulus and traveling toward the septum, ending in the aortomitral continuity (**Fig. 3**). The LVA communicated with atrial branches and with branches posterior to the aortic root. LVA communicated via collateral flow with the LVS septal veins in 11 of 19 patients (58%)

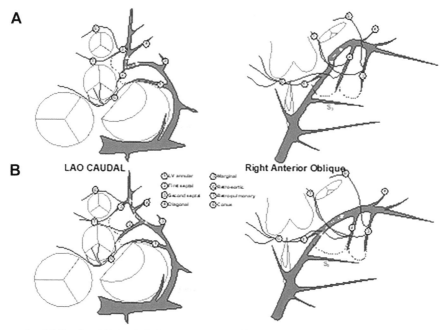

Fig. 2. Schematic of LVS veins. (*A*) Angled GCV–AIV junction. (*B*) Nonangled GCV–AIV junction. LAO caudal is best to display the sequence of LVS veins, whereas RAO foreshortens the LV annular vein and is best for AIV septals. LVS veins are labeled 1 to 8. See the text for details.

(see **Fig. 3**). In the left anterior oblique (LAO) projection, the LVA vein coursed more septal than the AIV, toward the aortomitral continuity, giving posterior branches to the left atrium and anterior branches toward the AIV septal vein, which overlapped in this projection (**Fig. 4**F). In the right anterior oblique (RAO) projection, the LVA was completely foreshortened (**Fig. 4**) and overlapping the GCV, and only its retroaortic/atrial branches or collaterals to AIV septals were visible (see **Fig. 4**G). LVA cannulation with multielectrode catheters would typically contain atrial and ventricular signals (hence the "annular" denomination) (see **Fig. 4**C). The LVA contained arrhythmogenic substrate and was targeted for ethanol infusion in a minority (6/53 [11%]) of cases, with acute success in all six cases.[26]

Left ventricular septal veins

LVS septal veins: Defined as branches of the AIV that ran rightward and intramural to the interventricular groove. LV septal veins could arise as high as the GCV–AIV junction, and there typically were more than one. **Fig. 5** shows examples of their variability. A previous report labeled some LVS septal as LVS "communicating vein," a denomination that also included LVA veins.[23] LVS septal veins run rightward and deep in the septum (true "perforators") (see **Fig. 4**F). LVS septal veins arising at the GCV–AIV junction could connect with retroaortic branches and contain atrial signals, analogous to LVA veins, or with branches posterior to the RV outflow between the RVOT and LVOT. **Fig. 6** shows examples of two LVS septal veins illustrating their 3D relationships with neighboring structures. The first LVS septal had atrial and ventricular signals and was retroaortic (**Figs. 5**E and **6**A), whereas the second LVS septal ran anterior to the aorta and posterior to the RVOT (see **Fig. 6**F–K). More commonly, all LVS septals were located anterior to the aortic root (see **Fig. 6**) and not retroaortic (which was typical of LVA veins). LVS septals were present in all 53 venograms. The LVS septal was targeted for ethanol infusion in 38 of 53 cases, with success in 37 of 38 (97%).[26]

LVS diagonal veins. Defined as branches of the AIV that ran leftward to the interventricular groove. Diagonals can arise as high as the GCV–AIV junction. Diagonal veins were present in 51 of 53 venograms (96%). Examples are shown in **Fig. 5**L and M. Despite the near-consistent presence of LVS diagonal veins, they seldom harbored signals targeted for VEA. LVS diagonal veins were targeted, with success for ethanol infusion in 2 cases.[26]

Collateral flow. LVS veins commonly had collaterals communicating one another. LVA communicated with LVS septal veins in 11 of 19 (58%). LVS septal veins 1 and 2 also communicated with each other in 25 of 53 (47%) (see **Figs. 3**, **4**, and **6**).[26]

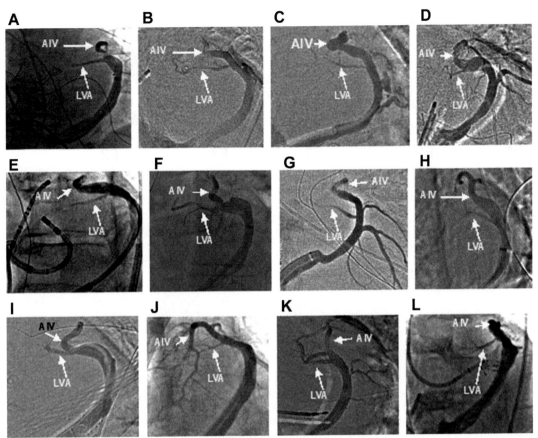

Fig. 3. LVA vein examples. (*A–L*) Examples of LVA shown in left anterior oblique, steep caudal projection. LVA arises from the GCV before the GCV–AIV transition, runs toward the septum, underneath the GCV–AIV junction, and toward the aortomitral continuity (see aortic valve prosthesis in *A*). Abbreviations as in **Fig. 2**.

Branches beyond LVS. Retroaortic branches to right atrium and conus branches. Retroaortic branches of either LVA veins or proximal LVS septal veins arising close to the GCV–AIV junction could extend posterior to the aorta and connect with veins draining in the right atrium. Typically, LVS septal ran anterior to the aorta and posterior to the RVOT, but an RVOT conus vein, anterior to the RVOT was seen in 7 of 53 cases.[26] See **Fig. 7**.

Procedure

Fluoroscopy
The veins are best visualized in LAO (30° to 45°), steep caudal (40° to 50°) fluoroscopic projection, analogous to the "spider view" used in coronary arteriography.

Relevance of left anterior oblique caudal projection
Angiographic images of LVS veins are challenging due to foreshortening and overlap. Most previous reports contain RAO views, [23–25] which are adequate for LVS septal veins arising from the AIV, but RAO foreshortens the GCV as it wraps around the mitral annulus toward the LVS, as well as LVA vein. Although RAO is useful to assess retroaortic versus retropulmonary vein courses, it has limited utility for vein selection. The LAO caudal is uniquely suited to display all LVS veins in their totality. The caudal angulation must be steep enough to display the AIV in an elongated fashion. Only then can the full spectrum of LVS veins be displayed at once.[26]

Coronary sinus access and preliminary mapping
In all procedures, efforts should be made to localize VT substrate within an area amenable to RFA. Electroanatomical maps (EAM) are constructed by using 3D mapping systems (NavX, St Jude Medical, St Paul, MN) or Carto3 (Biosense-Webster, Diamond Bar, CA). Mapping strategies include substrate maps to localize low-bipolar voltage areas in the presence of structural heart disease, activation maps and pace-maps. Access to the epicardial space via a subxiphoid anterior

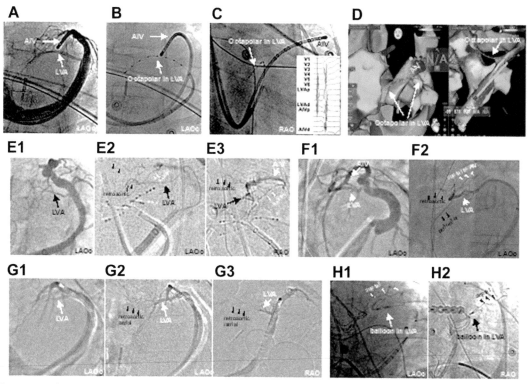

Fig. 4. Branching and 3D location of LVA vein. (*A–D*) LVA cannulated with an octapolar catheter, in left anterior oblique steep caudal (LAOc) projection (*A, B*). (*C*) In RAO projection, the LVA is foreshortened and basal, and contains atrial and ventricular signals (inset). (*D*) Incorporating LVA to the 3D map, LVA wraps around the mitral valve in LAO (*left*) and posterior to the aorta in LAO cranial view (*right*). (*E–H*) Nonselective (*e1, f1, g1, h1*) versus selective LVA venograms. Selective LVA venograms show retroaortic branches and collaterals to septal branches of the AIV, both seen in LAOc (*e2, f2, g2*) and RAO projections (*e3, g3*).

puncture can be undertaken when suitable for epicardial mapping and ablation.[17]

RCVEA is considered when: (1) RFA failed at the best endocardial sites as guided by the earliest activation or best pace-mapping (PM); (2) when feasible, epicardial RFA failed or was deemed not indicated due to proximity to coronary arteries or due to presence of the earliest activation site at a broad area; and (3) when optimal PM and/or earliest activation was obtained from within a coronary vein.[17]

Stable CS access is necessary. We perform coronary vein mapping by advancing a long 8F sheath in the CS via the right femoral vein (Preface, Biosense-Webster, Diamond Bar, CA) or via the right internal jugular vein (CPS sheath, St Jude Medical, Sylmar, CA). Coronary venograms are performed. A multipolar catheter is inserted in the CS and selected ventricular branches (4F quadripolar IBI, St Jude, or Deca-Nav, Biosense-Webster). A multipolar catheter is then inserted in the CS for local activation time and 3D electroanatomic maps (**Table 1**), although typically only the proximal AIV can be reached. Mapping methods

used include activation or pace-map correlation maps using 3D mapping systems (CARTO, Biosense Webster; or NavX, St Jude Medical). Most commonly, multielectrode catheters cannot penetrate small coronary veins, but they can indicate the earliest region around which to search penetrating intramyocardial branches (**Figs. 6**A–C and **7**A–C). Mapping and pacing from small coronary veins can also be performed by advancing an angioplasty wire (BMW 0.014″, Abbott), connected to an alligator clip in a unipolar configuration with a reference electrode as a needle inserted in the thigh skin. This approach leads to significantly reduced noise compared with using Wilson's central terminal or an indifferent electrode in the inferior vena cava, and provides exclusively local signals, compared with using a neighboring electrode. Selective wire cannulation of different targeted veins is achieved by introducing an LIMA angioplasty guide catheter and torquing it in the desired direction, or simply by guiding the angioplasty wire with the help of a torquing device. To obtain unipolar signals from selective portions of the targeted vein, the angioplasty balloon is

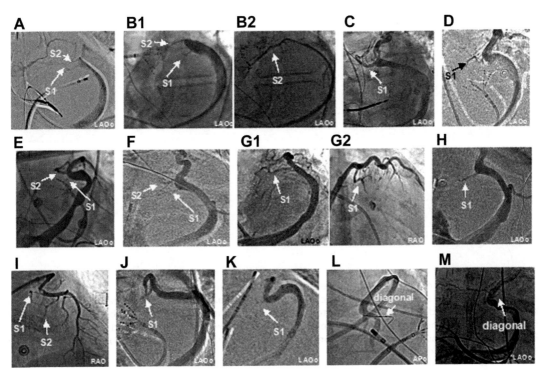

Fig. 5. LVS septal and diagonal veins. (*A–K*) Septal branches arise at the GCV–AIV junction (S1) and in the proximal AIV (S2). Typically more than one septal branch exist, with common collateral flow between them. In RAO (g2), septal veins are foreshortened compared with LAO. (*L–M*) Diagonal veins arising from the proximal AIV (*L*), shown in APc view, or from the GCV–AIV junction (*M*). Abbreviations as in **Fig. 3**.

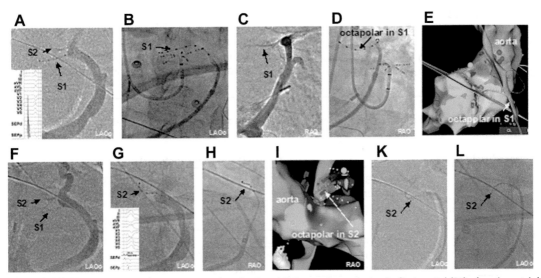

Fig. 6. 3D location of proximal GCV–AIV LVS septal veins. (*A*) Octapolar catheter in first septal (S1), showing atrial and ventricular signals (consecutive, proximal-to-distal septal bipolar signals SEPp-SEPd in the inset). (*B*) PentaRay catheter via retroaortic approach showing apparent overlap with octapolar. (*C–E*) Venogram and catheter positioning of S1 in RAO showing a posterior course relative to aorta, confirmed by 3D map from a left lateral view (*E*). (*F–L*) Cannulation of second septal (S2). Octapolar catheter in S2 (*G*) shows no atrial signals (inset) and an early signal in SEPd, which was targeted with ethanol. In RAO, octapolar catheter is foreshortened (*H*), but 3D map shows its course anterior to the aorta. (*J,K*) Selective venogram and balloon cannulation of S2. Abbreviations as in previous figures.

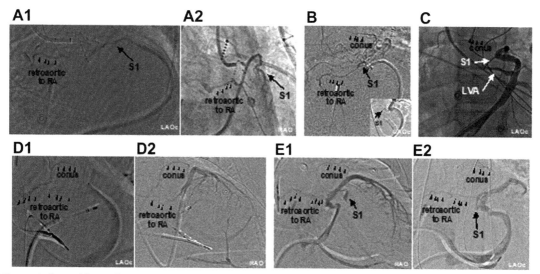

Fig. 7. Collateral flow of LVS veins. (*A, B*) Selective S1 venograms showing collateral flow to retroaortic branches eventually draining in the RA, shown in LAOc (*a1, b*) and in RAO (*a2*). Note that in RAO (*a2*), relative to the PentaRay catheter inserted in the aorta, S1 is anterior to the aorta, whereas the retroaortic branch is posterior to it. Inset in b shows a catheter in aorta for reference. (*C*) Collateral flow from LVA to S1, and conus branch draining into the RA. (*D–E*) Conus branch and retroaortic collaterals to RA, shown in LAOc (*d1, e1*) and RAO (*d2, e2*). Abbreviations as in previous figures.

advanced over the wire to cover it except for the most distal 3 to 5 mm, which acts as the active electrode.[27]

DEFINING TARGET VENULES

Once the earliest site in the GCV/AIV has been delineated, coronary venograms are performed to delineate the GCV, AIV, and small diagonal or septal (tributaries to assess suitable target branches that provide access to the targeted VT

substrate in the LVS). It is important to find the best fluoroscopic projection, which is highly variable. Balloon occlusion venograms are optimal, but not mandatory, for this purpose. For proximal LVS diagonal branches of the AIV, we use the LAO caudal view and for septal AIV branches, we use the RAO caudal view. Mapping, pacing, and selective cannulation of these branches are achieved by advancing an angioplasty guidewire (Balance Middleweight [BMW] 0.014 inches; Abbott, Santa Clara, CA) into the vessel with the

Table 1
Procedural steps and required equipment used in retrograde coronary venous ethanol ablation of ventricular

Procedural Step	Device (Size, Manufacturer)		
CS cannulation	Preface (Biosense Webster)	SL1 (Abbott)	Agilis (Abbott)
GCV/AIV mapping	DecaNav (7F, Biosense Webster)	INQUIRY (4- 0r 10-pole 4F; Abbott)	Map-iT (20-pole, 3.3 F; APT EP)
Guide catheter	LIMA guide	LIMA guide	LIMA guide
Wire mapping	BMW (o.014 inch, Abbott)	VisionWire (0.014 inch, Biotronik)	
Alligator clips	Threshold cable (Abbott)		
Selective ethanol infusion	OTW Sprinter Legend (1.25 to 2.5 × 6 mm; Medtronic)	Finecross (Terumo)	

Abbreviations: AIV, anterior interventricular vein; BMW, balance middleweight; CS, coronary sinus; GCV, great cardiac vein; LIMA, left internal mammary artery; OTW, over the wire.

help of an LIMA angioplasty guide catheter (Boston Scientific, Marlborough, MA) which adds stability and torqueability. An angioplasty balloon (typically 6 mm × 2 mm) is advanced over the wire except the most distal portion (approximately 3 mm of exposed angioplasty wire), which is configured as a unipolar electrode with an alligator clip. A specifically designed wire with an active distal electrode can be used (VisionWire, Biotronik, Berlin, Germany), otherwise, any electrically conductive wire can be used. We use a needle inserted in the groin skin as the reference electrode, but the Wilson central terminal or an inferior vena cava electrode can be used as well. Unipolar signals and pace maps can be used to confirm the candidacy of the targeted vein for ethanol ablation (see **Figs. 1** and **2**). If the targeted venule is tortuous, a Finecross microguide catheter (Finecross MG catheter, Terumo, Tokyo, Japan) can be used instead of the angioplasty balloon because it can follow the wire more readily.[27]

Ethanol Delivery

If wire signals support the adequacy of the cannulated vein as a target, the wire is then retracted, the angioplasty balloon is inflated, and contrast is injected in the targeted venule to assess its size and the extent of myocardial staining, which would indicate the tissue reached. It is important to recognize that no therapeutic effect is to be expected if the vein injected has collaterals back to the CS, bypassing myocardium, or if a large vein is injected and targeted signals are only present proximally in the vein. Initially, 1 cc of 96% to 98% ethanol (American Regent Inc, Shirley, NY; or Akorn Inc, Lake Forest, IL) is delivered. The angioplasty balloon remains inflated after ethanol infusion until the therapeutic response is assessed. A complete seal is not required because leaked ethanol is safely diluted by CS flow in the right atrium. Indeed, if the Finecross catheter is used, no venule occlusion ever occurs because it lacks a balloon.

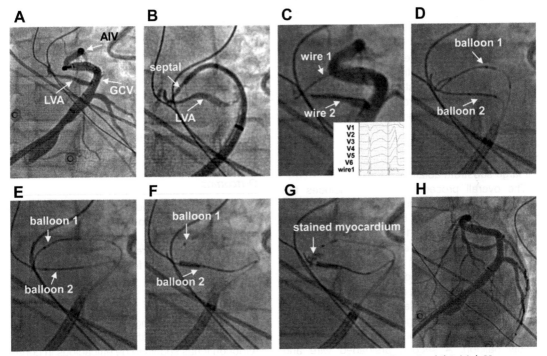

Fig. 8. Double-balloon technique to prevent collateral flow from septal to annular vein. (*A*) Initial CS venogram showing a large LVA vein, but the electrodes from the junction of the GCV with the AIV showed the best signals. (*B*) Venogram via a left internal mammary artery catheter showing a large septal vein at the GCV–AIV junction, with extensive collateral flow to the LVA. (*C*) Unipolar wire signal from the septal vein (wire 1) showed the best signals, preceding the QRS by 28 ms. A second wire was inserted into the LVA vein (wire 2). (*D*) Two angioplasty balloons were inserted over their respective wires. (*E*) Balloon 1 was positioned in the septal vein, where the best signal had been recorded, whereas balloon 2 was inserted in the LVA vein to block collateral flow. (*F*) Inflation of balloon 1. (*G*) After inflation of balloon 2, contrast injection in the septal vein via balloon 1 led to myocardial staining in the targeted location without collateral flow. This led to elimination of the extrasystoles. (*H*) Final CS venogram.

After contrast is injected in the targeted vessel and myocardial staining is verified, repeat 1 cc injection (up to 4) of ethanol over 2 min each. Myocardial staining is observed, and intracardiac echocardiograms show an area of increased echogenicity. In our experience, repeated injections are necessary to consolidate a therapeutic effect because myocardial tissue reached by retrograde venous ethanol may be compromised by competing for anterograde arterial flow.[27]

Determinants of ethanol success

For therapeutic success, ethanol must reach the targeted myocardium. Failures are to be expected if: (1) ethanol is delivered to the inappropriate target; or (2) ethanol does not reach the target. Meticulous mapping is required to select the appropriate vein located in the myocardium where VAs come from. Technical difficulties reaching the targeted vein with a stable catheter for ethanol delivery can be significant, because of the complex 3D architecture of the ventricular venous vasculature. Once cannulated, myocardial reach depends on the size of the injected vein, the extent of the capillary network associated with it, and the absence of collaterals that could shunt ethanol away from myocardium.[17] If the ablated vein allows, we typically will recannulate the targeted vein with a multipolar catheter. After cannulation, signals pre- and post-ethanol ablation are compared along with proof that the epicardium can no longer be captured with pacing.[20]

Double balloon technique

We have developed a double-balloon technique for large substrate ablation[28] (**Fig. 8**).

The overall procedure strategy includes the following steps, after identifying the targeted vein: (1) inflation of both balloons; (2) injection of contrast; (3) injection of 1 cc ethanol over 1 min; (4) injection of contrast to assess myocardial staining; (5) repeat injection of 1 cc ethanol (up to 4 per balloon positioning); and (6) balloon deflation, repositioning, and repeat injection as needed.[28]

Once early signals identify the optimal vein, contrast venography is again performed to assess collaterals. The wire is preloaded with an angioplasty balloon. A second preloaded wire and balloon is advanced in the vein as well. The targeted region of the vein is divided into segments. For each segment, a distal balloon (Sprinter 2.5 × 6 mm; Medtronic, Minneapolis, MN) is positioned and inflated at one end to occlude flow, leaving the wire in. The proximal balloon (Sprinter 2.75 × 6 mm; Medtronic) is positioned at the beginning of the segment and inflated. The wire of the proximal balloon is removed, and contrast

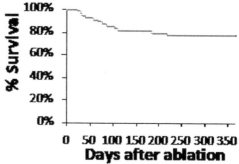

Fig. 9. Outcomes of RCVEA. In a series of previous radiofrequency ablation failures, ethanol ablation led to a 76% success at 1-year follow-up.

is injected via the proximal balloon to verify distal occlusion and show the extent of myocardial staining via small intramural vein branches between the two balloons. Then, 2 to 4 injections of 1 cc ethanol are delivered slowly over 2 min. Intracardiac echocardiography is used to monitor changes in myocardial local echogenicity, indicating ethanol penetration into the tissue. Contrast injection after ethanol shows increased tissue staining compared with the initial injection. The proximal balloon is then flushed, and the balloons are deflated and moved into more proximal portions of the vein. Sequentially, multiple positionings are used to deliver ethanol along the targeted portion of the vein (see **Fig. 8**).[28]

Outcomes

RCVEA was developed as a "bailout" approach, and thus, there are no randomized comparisons with other approaches. In our series of 53 patients, we obtained a 76% freedom from ventricular arrhythmias at 1 year of follow-up (**Fig. 9**).

SUMMARY

Chemical ablation using the transcoronary arterial system has a lengthy but arduous history. Although it has shown to be efficacious in controlling VAs, safety concerns from cannulation of the coronary arterial system to unwanted ethanol downstream effects, have limited TCEA's use. RCVEA has shown promising results. Although it appears to be in its infancy, RCVEA appears to be the future of chemical ablation in comparison to TCEA due to its increased safety and efficacy. Prospective randomized trial data are needed for this adjunctive treatment to RFA.

CLINICS CARE POINTS

- Ventricular venous ethanol can be useful to treat ablation-refractory arrhythmias.

SOURCES OF FUNDING

This study was supported by the Charles Burnett III and Lois and Carl Davis Centennial Chair endowments (Houston, Texas, USA).

REFERENCES

1. Baker RC, Kramer RE. Cytotoxicity of short-chain alcohols. Annu Rev Pharmacol Toxicol 1999;39:127–50.
2. Lasner M, Roth LG, Chen CH. Structure-functional effects of a series of alcohols on acetylcholinesterase-associated membrane vesicles: elucidation of factors contributing to the alcohol action. Arch Biochem Biophys 1995;317:391–6.
3. Lenaz G, Parenti-Castelli G, Sechi AM. Lipid-protein interactions in mitochondria. Changes in mitochondrial adenosine triphosphatase activity induced by n-butyl alcohol. Arch Biochem Biophys 1975;167:72–9.
4. Das AM, Harris DA. Regulation of the mitochondrial ATP synthase is defective in rat heart during alcohol-induced cardiomyopathy. Biochim Biophys Acta 1993;1181:295–9.
5. Auffermann W, Camacho SA, Wu S, et al. 31P and 1H magnetic resonance spectroscopy of acute alcohol cardiac depression in rats. Magn Reson Med 1988;8:58–69.
6. Schurmann P, Penalver J, Valderrabano M. Ethanol for the treatment of cardiac arrhythmias. Curr Opin Cardiol 2015;30:333–43.
7. Hammer FD, Boon LM, Mathurin P, et al. Ethanol sclerotherapy of venous malformations: evaluation of systemic ethanol contamination. J Vasc Interv Radiol 2001;12:595–600.
8. Chilson DA, Peigh PS, Mahomed Y, et al. Chemical ablation of ventricular tachycardia in the dog. Am Heart J 1986;111:1113–8.
9. Inoue H, Waller BF, Zipes DP. Intracoronary ethyl alcohol or phenol injection ablates aconitine-induced ventricular tachycardia in dogs. J Am Coll Cardiol 1987;10:1342–9.
10. Brugada P, de Swart H, Smeets JL, et al. Transcoronary chemical ablation of ventricular tachycardia. Circulation 1989;79:475–82.
11. Kay GN, Epstein AE, Bubien RS, et al. Intracoronary ethanol ablation for the treatment of recurrent sustained ventricular tachycardia. J Am Coll Cardiol 1992;19:159–68.
12. Haines DE, Whayne JG, DiMarco JP. Intracoronary ethanol ablation in swine: effects of ethanol concentration on lesion formation and response to programmed ventricular stimulation. J Cardiovasc Electrophysiol 1994;5:422–31.
13. Kumar S, Barbhaiya CR, Sobieszczyk P, et al. Role of alternative interventional procedures when endo- and epicardial catheter ablation attempts for ventricular arrhythmias fail. Circ Arrhythm Electrophysiol 2015;8:606–15.
14. Sacher F, Sobieszczyk P, Tedrow U, et al. Transcoronary ethanol ventricular tachycardia ablation in the modern electrophysiology era. Heart Rhythm 2008;5:62–8.
15. Tokuda M, Sobieszczyk P, Eisenhauer AC, et al. Transcoronary ethanol ablation for recurrent ventricular tachycardia after failed catheter ablation: an update. Circ Arrhythm Electrophysiol 2011;4:889–96.
16. Wright KN, Morley T, Bicknell J, et al. Retrograde coronary venous infusion of ethanol for ablation of canine ventricular myocardium. J Cardiovasc Electrophysiol 1998;9:976–84.
17. Kreidieh B, Rodriguez-Manero M, P AS, et al. Retrograde coronary venous ethanol infusion for ablation of refractory ventricular tachycardia. Circ Arrhythm Electrophysiol 2016;9. https://doi.org/10.1161/CIRCEP.116.004352e004352.
18. Baldinger SH, Kumar S, Barbhaiya CR, et al. Epicardial radiofrequency ablation failure during ablation procedures for ventricular arrhythmias: reasons and implications for outcomes. Circ Arrhythm Electrophysiol 2015;8:1422–32.
19. Baher A, Shah DJ, Valderrabano M. Coronary venous ethanol infusion for the treatment of refractory ventricular tachycardia. Heart Rhythm 2012;9:1637–9.
20. Tavares L, Lador A, Fuentes S, et al. Intramural venous ethanol infusion for refractory ventricular arrhythmias. Outcomes of a multicenter experience. J Am Coll Cardiol EP 2020. https://doi.org/10.1016/j.jacep.2020.07.023.
21. Loukas M, Bilinsky S, Bilinsky E, et al. Cardiac veins: a review of the literature. Clin Anat 2009;22:129–45.
22. Bai W, Xu X, Ma H, et al. Assessment of the relationship between the coronary venous and arterial systems using 256-slice computed tomography. J Comput Assist Tomogr 2020;44:1–6.
23. Komatsu Y, Nogami A, Shinoda Y, et al. Idiopathic ventricular arrhythmias originating from the vicinity of the communicating vein of cardiac venous systems at the left ventricular summit. Circ Arrhythm Electrophysiol 2018;11:e005386.
24. Yokokawa M, Good E, Chugh A, et al. Intramural idiopathic ventricular arrhythmias originating in the

intraventricular septum: mapping and ablation. Circ Arrhythm Electrophysiol 2012;5:258–63.

25. Briceno DF, Enriquez A, Liang JJ, et al. Septal coronary venous mapping to guide substrate characterization and ablation of intramural septal ventricular arrhythmia. JACC Clin Electrophysiol 2019;5: 789–800.

26. Tavares L, Fuentes S, Lador A, et al. Venous anatomy of the left ventricular summit: therapeutic implications for ethanol infusion. Heart Rhythm 2021;18:1557–65.

27. Tavares L, Valderrabano M. Retrograde venous ethanol ablation for ventricular tachycardia. Heart Rhythm 2019;16:478–83.

28. Da-Wariboko A, Lador A, Tavares L, et al. Double-balloon technique for retrograde venous ethanol ablation of ventricular arrhythmias in the absence of suitable intramural veins. Heart Rhythm 2020;17: 2126–34.

Fluoroless Catheter Ablation of Left Ventricular Summit Arrhythmias
A Step-by-Step Approach

Jorge Romero, MD, FHRS[a], Juan Carlos Diaz, MD[b], Maria Gamero, MD[a],
Isabella Alviz, MD[a], Marta Lorente, MD[a], Mohamed Gabr, MD[a],
Cristian Camilo Toquica, MD[a], Suraj Krishnan, MD[a], Alejandro Velasco, MD[a],
Aung Lin, MD[a], Andrea Natale, MD, FHRS[c], Fengwei Zou, MD[a],
Luigi Di Biase, MD, PhD, FHRS[a],*

KEYWORDS

- Fluoroless • Cardiac ablation • Idiopathic ventricular arrythmias • Radiation
- Intracardiac echocardiography • Electroanatomic mapping

KEY POINTS

- Use of fluoroscopy guidance for catheter ablation is associated with risks secondary to radiation exposure and the use of lead.
- Fluoroless catheter ablation can be safely and effectively performed, thus averting these risks.
- Ablation of ventricular arrhythmias arising from the left ventricular summit is feasible with proper knowledge of cardiac anatomy and familiarity with intracardiac ultrasound and electroanatomic mapping.

INTRODUCTION

Idiopathic ventricular arrythmias (VAs) originating from the left ventricular (LV) summit are relatively frequent, accounting for 10% to 15% of all VAs.[1] Given the low efficacy of different drugs to suppress these arrhythmias, catheter ablation (CA) has established itself as the mainstay treatment. Noteworthy, the intricate anatomic relationships involving different areas such as the LV outflow tract (LVOT), right ventricular outflow tract (RVOT), sinuses of Valsalva (SoV), aortomitral continuity (AMC), coronary arteries, and cardiac veins [including the coronary sinus (CS) great cardiac vein (GCV), and anterior interventricular vein (AIV)] pose a challenge even for expert operators (**Fig. 1**). Therefore, it is indispensable for electrophysiologists, particularly those in training, to acquire in-depth knowledge of the cardiac anatomy and mastering different imaging modalities.[2]

Despite the use of intracardiac echocardiography (ICE) and electroanatomic mapping (EAM) systems to confirm catheter position and movement, fluoroscopy persists as the sine qua non-component of CA for most electrophysiologists. However, prolonged fluoroscopy use can result in hazardous exposure to ionizing radiation with subsequent detrimental effects for patients,

[a] Montefiore Medical Center, Albert Einstein College of Medicine, Bronx, NY, USA; [b] Arrhythmia and electrhophysiology service, Clinica Las Vegas, Grupo Quiron Salud; Universidad CES School of Medicine, Medellin, Colombia, USA; [c] Texas Cardiac Arrhythmia Institute, St. David's Medical Center, Austin, TX, USA
* Corresponding author. Montefiore Medical Center, Albert Einstein College of Medicine, 111 East 210th Street, Bronx, NY 10467.
E-mail address: dibbia@gmail.com

Card Electrophysiol Clin 15 (2023) 75–83
https://doi.org/10.1016/j.ccep.2022.10.002
1877-9182/23/© 2023 Elsevier Inc. All rights reserved.

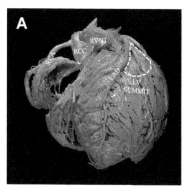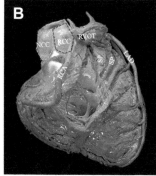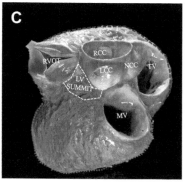

Fig. 1. Anatomical relations between adjacent and opposing structures within the LV summit (*yellow dashed line*). (*A*) Given the proximity between the LV summit and the coronary arteries, ablation from within the GCV/AIV (which would be located at the base of the dashed triangle delineating the LV summit) increases the risk of the coronary lesion. (*B*) Relation between the RVOT, the LV summit, and the LAD artery. In some cases, ablation from within the most leftward portion of the RVOT can be used to target arrhythmias arising from the LV summit. However, operators should be aware that the LAD artery lies near the RVOT and could be injured during prolonged RF applications. (*C*) Relation between the LV summit, the sinuses of Valsalva (ie, LCC and RCC) and the RVOT. GCV/AIV, great cardiac vein/anterior interventricular vein; LAD, left anterior descending; LCC, left coronary cusp; LV, left ventricle; MV, mitral valve; NCC, noncoronary cusp; RCA, right coronary artery; RCC, right coronary cusp; RF, radiofrequency; RVOT, right ventricular outflow tract; SP, septal perforator; TV, tricuspid valve; VAs, ventricular arrhythmias. (*From* Romero J, Shivkumar K, Valderrabano M, et al. Modern mapping and ablation techniques to treat ventricular arrhythmias from the left ventricular summit and interventricular septum [published correction appears in Heart Rhythm. 2020 Sep 23;:]. Heart Rhythm. 2020;17(9):1609-1620; with permission.)

physicians, and other electrophysiology laboratory staff.[3–5] There are two types of injury patterns from exposure to ionizing radiation: (a) deterministic (ie, dose-dependent), which results in damage such as skin erythema and cataracts; and (b) stochastic (ie, non-dose dependent, which means there is no "safe threshold") which predisposes to genetic defects with subsequent malignancies and birth defects.[6,7] In general, radiation

exposure after ablation of VAs is between 8–25 mSv, equivalent to 6–28 computed tomography scans or 60–280 chest X-rays, representing an increased lifetime attributable risk of 60 to 80 excess cancers per 100,000 treated patients.[8] As a result, the risk of cataracts (4.7% vs 0.7%, $p = 0.003$), skin lesions (8.6% vs 2%, $p = 0.002$), and orthopedic illnesses from heavy protection equipment (30% vs 5.4%, $p < 0.001$)

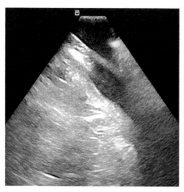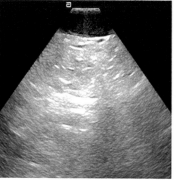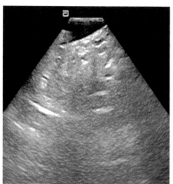

APPLY ANTERIOR DEFLECTION   ADVANCE   APPLY POSTERIOR DEFLECTION

Fig. 2. Tips for advancing the ICE catheter from the femoral vein to the right atrium. If an obtuse angle is observed (*left*), anterior deflection should be applied. Conversely, if an acute angle is observed in front of the catheter (*right*), gentle posterior deflection should be applied to align the catheter with the long axis of the vein. If the operator does not feel comfortable with advancing the ICE catheter without fluoroscopy, the use of long sheaths will facilitate navigation through the abdominal venous anatomy and deliver the ICE probe closer to the heart.

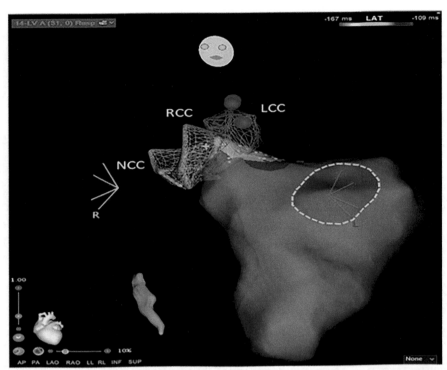

Fig. 3. Left ventricular shell created by merging information obtained from electroanatomic mapping and ICE images using the SoundStar system. The left (LCC), right (RCC) and noncoronary cusps (NCC) can be easily identified, along with the mitral valve annulus (*dotted line*) clearly delineating the aorto-mitral continuity (AMC). This reduces the amount of time needed to produce an anatomical map and reduces the need to rely on fluoroscopic imaging.

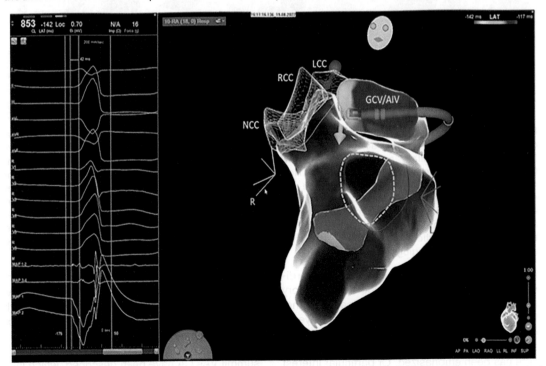

Fig. 4. Fluoroless electroanatomic mapping showing the intimate relationship between different anatomical structures. Although the GCV/AIV has a clearly early activation (−42 ms), to perform ablation from within the GCV/AIV a coronary angiogram is usually needed, thus requiring the use of fluoroscopy. Instead, ablation can be performed from within opposing structures, such as the infravalvular LCC or the AMC. AIV, anterior interventricular vein; AMC, aorto mitral continuity; GCV, great cardiac vein; LCC, left coronary cusp; NCC, noncoronary cusp; RCC, right coronary cusp.

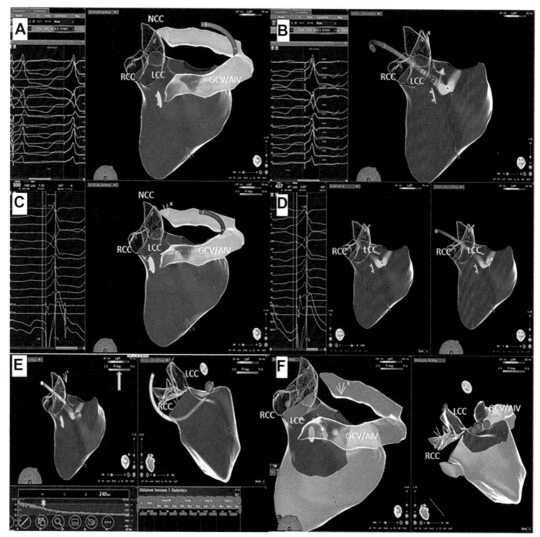

Fig. 5. Importance of evaluating adjacent structures. (*A*) A nearly perfect pace-map (99% match, red oval) was obtained from the GCV/AIV. (*B*) Pace mapping from the below the LCC shows less QRS similarity with the PVC (91.5% QRS match). Similarly, activation map from within the CS (*C*) shows earlier activation (−23 ms) than the (*D*) local activation time below the LCC (−5 ms). However, ablation was successful below the LCC (*E*). Note the marked impedance drop (yellow star) and the ablation settings (dashed rectangle): RF application lasted 4 min, with an average force of 13 g, power of 40 W and a marked impedance drop (43 Ω). During ablation, we prefer to use an impedance-based marker (*yellow arrow*), so that a drop >10 Ω can be visualized easily as a change in color from light pink to bright red. (*F*) The final lesion set is shown, showing the close relation between the GCV/AIV earliest site and the final ablation site. By performing ablation from the opposite structure, the need for coronary angiography is eliminated.

in health care personnel (eg, interventional cardiologists, cardiac electrophysiologists, laboratory nurses, and technicians) is significantly higher than in unexposed staff after a median of 10 years of exposure.[9] Hence, the importance of implementing techniques that reduce radiation exposure has been emphasized. Of particular interest is fluoroless CA, which was introduced more than a decade ago,[10] with fluoroless procedures routinely performed for ablation of supraventricular arrythmias and noncomplex VAs.[11,12] Yet, in

complex VAs, prolonged fluoroscopy and coronary angiogram are regularly used before delivering radiofrequency (RF) energy, particularly when performing ablation at the junction between the GCV and the AIV.[13]

Interestingly, new fluoroless techniques for LV summit VAs CA have been described, which integrate EAM and ICE to identify and subsequently ablate with very high procedural success.[14,15] The safety and effectiveness of this strategy has been recently shown, with similar efficacy and

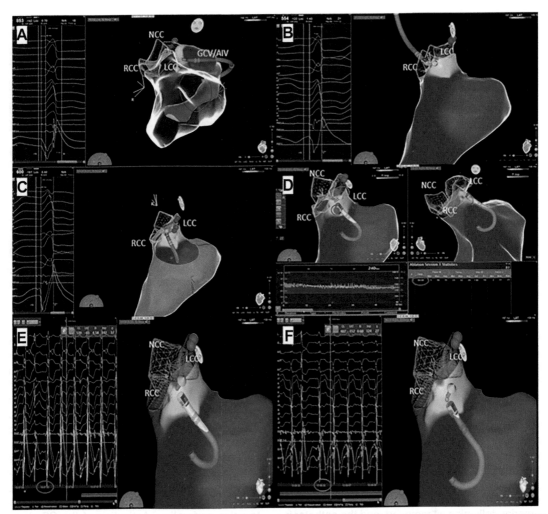

Fig. 6. (*A*) Early activation in the distal GCV/AIV (−42 ms). To avoid ablation from within the GCV/AIV, the LVOT was thoroughly mapped. (*B*) Activation mapping from within the RCC shows later activation (−7 ms) and the location is far from the earliest activation site within the GCV/AIV. (*C*) In the Right-left commissure below the valve, an area of early activation (−45 ms) is found, directly opposing the GCV/AIV early site. (*D*): long applications (4 min total; red oval) are required to achieve deep lesions to target the intramural site of origin. (*E*) The initial ablation lesion was performed during VT. (*F*) After approximately 35 s, VT terminated during ablation (*red circle*). However, ablation was continued for up to 4 min to ensure the elimination of an intramural focus.

safety for LV summit VAs using fluoroless CA compared with conventional fluoroscopic procedures.[16]

Thus, increasing knowledge and familiarity with ICE imaging and EAM, as well as training with fluoroless techniques can prepare electrophysiologists to abandon conventional fluoroscopy-guided CA procedures.

Step-by-Step Approach for Fluoroless Left Ventricular Summit Arrhythmia Ablation

Procedure setup and mapping technique
As previously stated, thorough understanding of the anatomy of the LVOT and RVOT, along with the anatomy of the aorta, coronary arteries, and

cardiac veins, is fundamental. We refer the reader to previous articles dedicated to anatomy.[1,2]

Under light sedation, percutaneous femoral venous and arterial access are obtained using the modified Seldinger technique under vascular ultrasound guidance. After obtaining vascular access, an ICE probe is advanced into the mid-right atrium (RA) with a careful manipulation of the ICE probe. Experienced operators can easily achieve this by maintaining an echo-free (black) area ahead of the transducer (**Fig. 2**). Less-experienced operators can rely on the use of long sheaths, which will enable the ICE probe to be delivered close to the heart. Entering the heart is easier when the probe is facing posteriorly (ie,

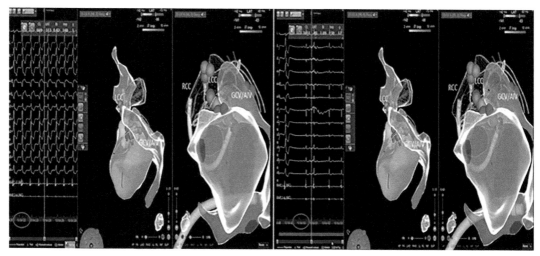

Fig. 7. Ablation during VT (*left*) frequently leads to early arrhythmia termination (*right*). However, ablation should be continued so that an intramural site of origin can be eliminated. As such, 3 to 4 min of RF application can be necessary to ensure arrhythmia elimination.

with the descending aorta in view). Once in the mid-RA, the probe is rotated counterclockwise (to approximately the 2 o'clock position) so that the tricuspid valve and the right ventricular (RV) inflow and outflow tract are observed. This is called home view. From this view, clockwise rotation of the ICE probe will reveal the aortic valve and the ascending aorta in a long-axis view (a slight posterior deflection may be needed). To observe the aortic valve in a short axis, the catheter is gently advanced into the RV after applying anterior deflection while on home view. Once in the RV, the anterior deflection es removed, and the catheter is gently rotated clockwise until the aorta is in view; slight rightward deflection is frequently needed to align the ICE view with the short axis. When using the SoundStar ICE catheter (Biosense Webster), a three-dimensional (3D) reconstruction of the different structures of both the RV and LVOT can be created and inserted into the mapping system. The surrounding anatomical areas such as the pulmonary valve, SoV, and the left and right coronary arteries are also visualized via CARTOSOUND. A detailed 3D shell is finally obtained after merging these 2D clips in different planes (**Fig. 3**).

For mapping and pacing, a 7-Fr deflectable catheter is advanced into the CS. To guide the placement of the CS catheter, two views of the heart right anterior oblique (RAO) and left anterior oblique (LAO) are displayed on the EAM system and the ostium of the CS is imaged with ICE. Once in the CS, the catheter is advanced to the GCV/AIV.[1,17]

Once the CS catheter is in place, a contact force-enabled ablation catheter is advanced through the femoral arterial access. Although the use of high-density mapping catheters (Pentarray, Biosense Webster or Advisor HD Grid, Abbott) is tempting, manipulation of these catheters is difficult in space-restricted areas (such as the distal CS, GCV, and AIV) and can lead to frequent ectopy that limit mapping efforts. The coronary cusps should be carefully mapped, delineating the anatomy as well as simultaneously performing activation mapping of the premature ventricular contraction (PVC) being careful not to exert excessive pressure on the aortic valve, as this can lead to valve perforation. Activation of the CS should also be annotated, with particular attention to the GCV/AIV area. Following supravalvular mapping, the catheter should be withdrawn into the descending aorta and curved into a J shape; curving catheters in the descending aorta reduces catheter manipulation in the aortic arch that could result in procedural complications including perforation and plaque embolization. Use of a long sheath is suggested to facilitate catheter manipulation, particularly in patients with tortuous arteries. The J-curve allows the catheters to advance through the aortic valve without the risk of valve perforation; this can be facilitated by viewing the ascending aorta in a long view. Once inside the LV, mapping should continue in the subaortic region and aorto mitral continuity (AMC). When performing activation mapping, it is important to underscore that a single-site PVC origin has an activation time greater than 30 ms pre-QRS, whereas a multiple-site PVC is defined as several "early" activation sites with a maximum pre-QRS activation time less than 30 ms.[14]

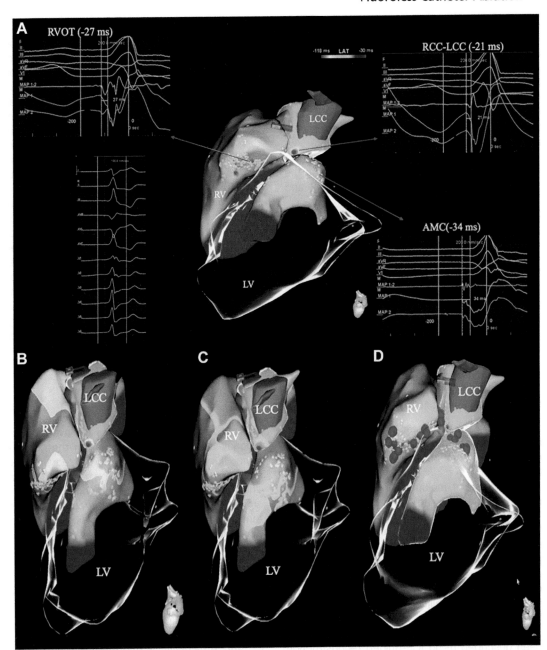

Fig. 8. Electroanatomic and activation mapping showing multiple sites for early activation in a patient with LVOT PVC. (*A*) Note similar activation times in the RVOT, RCC–LCC commissure, and AMC suggesting intramyocardial focus located in the area between these structures (LVS). *B* and *C*: Activation from this intramural focus is responsible for the similar activation times in different areas. D: By ablating from all these early points, the intramural focus is eliminated and a higher success rate is achieved.

Ablation technique

Different ablation settings (including power, contact force, and RF application duration) have been described depending on the area to be targeted. Using a conventional fluoroscopy approach, a coronary angiogram is frequently needed to determine the distance between the ablation point and the coronary vessels, adding time, radiation, and complexity to the procedure.

This is particularly true for arrhythmias originating in the GCV/AIV junction, since close proximity to the coronary arteries, the presence of thick adipose tissue, and the high baseline impedances frequently impede ablation. Indeed, in up to 75% of cases, RF energy is precluded in this region given that the coronary arteries are within 5 mm of GCV/AIV, and even at a distance >5 mm and <10 mm, coronary spasm has been described.

As such, fluoroless ablation of directly anatomically opposed structures (coronary cusps, LV subaortic region, AMC, and most leftward aspect of RVOT) without the need for ablation within the GCV/AIV (eliminating the need for coronary angiography) is feasible (**Fig. 4**).[18,19] Thus, to perform fluoroless CA of LV summit arrhythmias, we recommend:

1. Thorough mapping of the LVOT, including the coronary cusps, the infravalvular region, and the GCV/AIV.
2. Avoiding ablation from within the GCV/AIV by performing ablation in opposing or adjacent structures (thus eliminating the need for coronary angiography) (**Fig. 5**).
3. Using of 35 to 50 W of power while maintaining a contact force of 10 to 20 g.
4. Delivering long RF applications (up to 3–4 min each), even if the clinical arrhythmia disappears after a few seconds (**Figs. 6** and **7**). Use of prolonged RF applications to eliminate intramural LV summit arrhythmias relies on passive heat conduction from the area immediately underneath the catheter tip to adjacent areas.[20,21]
5. Aiming for at least 15 Ω of impedance drop.

Using this approach, procedural success can be achieved despite later local activation and poorer pace-map as compared with the best CS activation time.

In the case of multiple early activation areas (with all sites having an earliest activation <30 ms), CA is delivered sequentially, without following any particular order, in these anatomical sites irrespective of whether the clinical VA is suppressed or not (**Fig. 8**).[14] The presence of multiple areas indicates multiple exits from an intramyocardial focus, and ablation from different areas will have higher possibilities to reach the deeply located site of origin.

Although ablation from within the GCV/AIV has been described using ICE-guided reconstruction of the left main (LM) and proximal left anterior descending artery (LADA),[15] we recommend against this approach as inappropriate imaging of the LM can lead to inadequate representation of its location in the anatomical map and inadvertent RF application in its vicinity. Moreover, with our proposed approach the need for ablation from within the GCV/AIV can be eliminated.

CLINICAL OUTCOMES

Although fluoroless ablation is currently the standard of care in many centers for the management of supraventricular tachycardias and pulmonary vein isolation for atrial fibrillation ablation, the use of a fluoroless approach for the management of LV summit VAs is still uncommon. This could be related to the anatomical complexity of this area, which forces operators to rely on fluoroscopy, as well as a perceived higher risk of procedural complications or lower success rate. However, recent data have shown the safety and effectiveness of a fluoroless approach in this area. Rivera and colleagues[15] showed a procedure successful rate of 84% using an ICE-guided fluoroless technique for CA of LV summit VA, and a long-term freedom from VA recurrence of 76%. Likewise, a study comparing both techniques (with and without fluoroscopy) by Romero with by our Group[16] showed similar efficacy of fluoroless LV CA, with a procedural success rate of 87.5% in zero-fluoroscopy compared with 88% in fluoroscopy CA, and no major difference at 12-month follow-up (84% vs 81%) freedom from VA recurrence, respectively. Importantly, the safety of the fluoroless approach was evidenced by a similar risk of procedure-related complications.

SUMMARY

LV summit VA ablation without fluoroscopy is a feasible technique that appears to have a similar efficacy and safety compared with the conventional fluoroscopic procedure. By reducing the exposure to ionizing radiation, both the patient and the electrophysiology personnel can obtain significant benefits from this approach. It is important for the training electrophysiologist to be acquainted with these techniques.

CLINICS CARE POINTS

- Fluoroless ablation of arrhythmias arising from the LV summit can be performed safely and effectively, with no significant differences in outcomes compared to fluoroscopy-guided ablation.
- Thorough mapping is key to success of this technique.
- Ablation from within the GCV/AIV should be avoided so as to avoid the need for coronary angiography and inadvertently RF application in the vicinity of the LM/LAD coronaries.

DISCLOSURE

Dr L. Di Biase is a consultant for Stereotaxis, Biosense Webster, Boston Scientific, Abbott Medical, and has received speaker honoraria/travel from Medtronic, Atricure, Bristol Meyers Squibb, Pfizer, and Biotronik. Dr A. Natale is a consultant for Biosense Webster, Stereotaxis, Abbott, and has received speaker honoraria/travel from Medtronic, Atricure, Biotronik, and Janssen. The remaining authors report no conflict of interest.

REFERENCES

1. Yamada T, McElderry HT, Doppalapudi H, et al. Idiopathic ventricular arrhythmias originating from the left ventricular summit: anatomic concepts relevant to ablation. Circ Arrhythm Electrophysiol 2010;3(6): 616–23.

2. Romero J, Shivkumar K, Valderrabano M, et al. Modern mapping and ablation techniques to treat ventricular arrhythmias from the left ventricular summit and interventricular septum. Heart Rhythm 2020; 17(9):1609–20.

3. Lindsay BD, Eichling JO, Ambos HD, et al. Radiation exposure to patients and medical personnel during radiofrequency catheter ablation for supraventricular tachycardia. Am J Cardiol 1992;70:218–23.

4. Kovoor P, Ricciardello M, Collins L, et al. Risk to patients from radiation associated with radiofrequency ablation for supraventricular tachycardia. Circulation 1998;98:1534–40.

5. Perisinakis K, Damilakis J, Theocharopoulos N, et al. Accurate assessment of patient effective radiation dose and associated detriment risk from radiofrequency catheter ablation procedures. Circulation 2001;104:58–62.

6. Mahesh M. Fluoroscopy: patient radiation exposure issues. Radiographics 2001;21:1033–45.

7. Klein LW, Miller DL, Balter S, et al. Occupational health hazards in the interventional laboratory: time for a safer environment. Radiology 2009;250:538–44.

8. Casella M, Dello Russo A, Russo E, et al. X-ray exposure in cardiac electrophysiology: a retrospective analysis in 8150 patients over 7 Years of activity in a modern, large-volume laboratory. J Am Heart Assoc 2018;7(11):e008233.

9. Andreassi MG, Piccaluga E, Guagliumi G, et al. Occupational health risks in cardiac catheterization laboratory workers. Circ Cardiovasc interventions 2016;9:e003273.

10. Ferguson JD, Helms A, Mangrum JM, et al. Catheter ablation of atrial fibrillation without fluoroscopy using intracardiac echocardiography and electroanatomic mapping. Circ Arrhythm Electrophysiol 2009;2:611–9.

11. Razminia M, Willoughby MC, Demo H, et al. Fluoroless catheter ablation of cardiac arrhythmias: a 5-year experience. Pacing Clin Electrophysiol 2017; 40:425–33.

12. Sánchez JM, Yanics MA, Wilson P, et al. Fluoroless catheter ablation in adults: a single center experience. J Interv Card Electrophysiol 2016;45:199–207.

13. Enriquez A, Malavassi F, Saenz LC, et al. How to map and ablate left ventricular summit arrhythmias. Heart rhythm : official J Heart Rhythm Soc 2017; 14:141–8.

14. Di Biase L, Romero J, Zado ES, et al. Variant of ventricular outflow tract ventricular arrhythmias requiring ablation from multiple sites: intramural origin. Heart Rhythm 2019;16:724–32.

15. Rivera S, Vecchio N, Ricapito P, et al. Non-fluoroscopic catheter ablation of arrhythmias with origin at the summit of the left ventricle. J Interv Card Electrophysiol 2019;56:279–90.

16. Romero J, Velasco A, Díaz JC, et al. Fluoroless versus conventional mapping and ablation of ventricular arrhythmias arising from the left ventricular summit and interventricular septum. Circ Arrhythm Electrophysiol 2022;15:e010547.

17. Yamada T, Doppalapudi H, Maddox WR, et al. Prevalence and electrocardiographic and electrophysiological characteristics of idiopathic ventricular arrhythmias originating from intramural foci in the left ventricular outflow tract. Circ Arrhythm Electrophysiol 2016;9:e004079.

18. Jauregui Abularach ME, Campos B, Park KM, et al. Ablation of ventricular arrhythmias arising near the anterior epicardial veins from the left sinus of Valsalva region: ECG features, anatomic distance, and outcome. Heart rhythm : official J Heart Rhythm Soc 2012;9:865–73.

19. Nagashima K, Choi EK, Lin KY, et al. Ventricular arrhythmias near the distal great cardiac vein: challenging arrhythmia for ablation. Circ Arrhythm Electrophysiol 2014;7:906–12.

20. Garg L, Daubert T, Lin A, et al. Utility of prolonged duration endocardial ablation for ventricular arrhythmias originating from the left ventricular summit. JACC Clin Electrophysiol 2022;8:465–76.

21. Romero J, Ajijola OA, Boyle N, et al. Prolonged high-power endocardial ablation of epicardial microreentrant VT from the LV summit in a patient with nonischemic cardiomyopathy. HeartRhythm case Rep 2015;1:464–8.

Outcomes of Catheter Ablation of Left Ventricular Summit Arrhythmias

Abigail Louise D. Te-Rosano, MD[a,b,1], Fa-Po Chung, MD, PhD[a,c,*,1], Yenn-Jiang Lin, MD, PhD[a,c], Shih-Ann Chen, MD[a,d]

KEYWORDS

- Left ventricular summit • Ablation outcomes • Ventricular arrhythmia • Catheter ablation
- Percutaneous epicardial ablation • Ablation techniques

KEY POINTS

- Knowledge of the anatomic relationship between the left ventricular summit (LVS) and adjacent structures is important in mapping and ablation of ventricular arrhythmias (VA).
- A multicenter collaborative study demonstrated that acute success using the standard ablation approach for LVS VA was 82%, with long-term freedom from VA recurrence of 84%. LVS VS requiring multisite ablation was associated with higher VA recurrence.
- A percutaneous epicardial approach, such as bipolar ablation of 2 adjacent anatomic sites or retrograde coronary venous ethanol ablation, may be considered when successful elimination of LVS VA could not be achieved from the coronary venous system and/or adjacent sites.

INTRODUCTION

Catheter ablation is a well-established treatment strategy for patients with ventricular arrhythmia (VA). Although it is an effective and successful method, it has a variable success rate in treating epicardial and midmyocardial VA.[1] More than 12% of left VA arise from the epicardial surface of the left ventricle (LV),[2] and the left ventricular summit (LVS) is the most common site of origin. Recent studies have demonstrated the importance of LVS as the source of VAs, and a detailed and individualized characterization of the topographical relationship of adjacent structures to

the LVS region has substantial clinical implications in the approach to mapping and ablation of these arrhythmias.[2] LVS VAs are often targeted from the coronary venous system through the great cardiac vein/anterior interventricular vein (GCV/AIV), and because the origin could also be intramural below the epicardial LVS, they can also be approached via adjacent structures, such as the left coronary cusp (LCC), left ventricular outflow tract (LVOT) endocardium, or the septal right ventricular outflow tract (RVOT).[3–6] Furthermore, the right-left aortic interleaflet triangle located underneath the junction of the right and left commissure along the LV ostium is another anatomic vantage

Conflict of interest: None declared.

[a] Heart Rhythm Center and Division of Cardiology, Department of Medicine, Taipei Veterans General Hospital, No. 201, Sec. 2, Shih-Pai Road, Taipei, Taiwan; [b] HB Calleja Heart and Vascular Institute, St. Luke's Medical Center, 279 E. Rodriguez Sr. Avenue, Quezon City 1112, Philippines; [c] Department of Medicine, National Yang Ming Chiao Tung University, School of Medicine, Taipei, Taiwan; [d] Cardiovascular Center, Taichung Veterans General Hospital, Taichung, Taiwan

[1] These authors contributed equally to this work.

* Corresponding author. Heart Rhythm Center and Division of Cardiology, Department of Medicine, Taipei Veterans General Hospital, No. 201, Sec. 2, Shih-Pai Road, Taipei, Taiwan.

E-mail address: marxtaiji@gmail.com

Card Electrophysiol Clin 15 (2023) 85–92
https://doi.org/10.1016/j.ccep.2022.07.003

point from the endocardial anterior LV ostium for ablation of LVS VA.[7] Enriquez and colleagues[3] proposed a practical, comprehensive stepwise approach to mapping and ablation of VAs from the LVS using various adjacent structures as vantage points. A percutaneous epicardial approach is attempted only when ablation from these vantage points is unsuccessful or technically impossible. However, this approach is often limited by the presence of thick epicardial fat and a prominent myocardium on the anteroseptal aspect of the LVOT that could impede the appropriate radiofrequency (RF) energy delivered to the target areas.[3–6] Furthermore, because the LVS region is bounded and close to the major coronary vessels, this does not always allow safe ablation.[2] The latter is often the major reason for failed ablation of LVS VA. When RF ablation can be performed, the acute and long-term success rate is modest at best.[8] In this article, the authors aim to review the spatial and anatomic relationship of the structures surrounding the LVS, which provides vantage points for ablation, and the acute and long-term outcomes of different ablation approaches in LVS VA ablation.

ANATOMIC CONSIDERATIONS

LVS was a term coined by McAlpine[9] in 1975 to refer to the most superior portion of the epicardial LV region located above the upper end of the anterior interventricular sulcus and the aortic portion of the LV ostium anterior to the aortic valve (**Fig. 1**). It is a triangular region with its apex directed superiorly toward the ostium of the left main coronary artery (LMCA) and starts at the point of bifurcation of the left anterior descending (LAD) artery and left circumflex (LCx) artery.[10] Its right margin is bounded by the anterior interventricular groove with the LAD artery and AIV, whereas the left margin is delineated by the left coronary groove with the LCx artery and the initial section of the GCV. The base of this triangular region is delineated by an arcuate line, with the radius of this arc as the distance from the bifurcation of the LMCA to the first septal perforator of the LAD. The size of the LVS area depends on the first septal perforator's distance.[11] Within this triangular region, the GCV transitions from the left atrioventricular groove to the anterior atrioventricular groove as the AIV. Communicating vein branches of the GCV course epicardially over the LV summit region, whereas the septal perforating branches of the GCV drain the intramural LVOT myocardium underneath the LV summit.

The coronary venous system, particularly the GCV, plays an important role in dividing the LVS

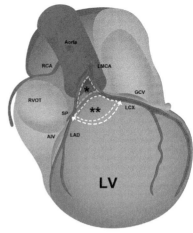

Fig. 1. The anatomic structure of LV summit. The LV summit is defined by the triangular region of the LV epicardium from the bifurcation between the LAD and LCx coronary arteries, and the base is generated by an arc connecting the first septal perforator branch (SP) of the LAD to the LCx (*white line* and *arrows*). The LV summit is separated into 2 regions according to the distribution of GCV and AIV. The upper portion at the apex of the triangle (*, *blue dotted line*) was considered inaccessible for epicardial approach owing to the presence of epicardial fat and adjacent to the coronary arteries, while lower portion of the triangle (**, *yellow dotted line*) was considered an accessible region for epicardial approach if successful ablation cannot be achieved from endocardial ablation. RCA, right coronary artery.

region into 2 clinically important areas. The superior area (also known as the basal LVS), which is an inaccessible area for conventional ablation, is triangular and dominates the inferior/accessible area in size.[4,11] The apex of this triangular region is closely related to the coronary vessels (LMCA and the bifurcation of LAD and LCx) and the aortic root, which is a continuation of the LVOT while deep into the myocardium. It is related to the left aortic sinus of Valsalva (LSOV), the septal summit to the right, and the aortomitral continuity to the left.[11] Epicardial lateral and septal sides of the inaccessible area are closely related to the left atrial appendage and the pulmonary trunk/RVOT, respectively,[11] and the base is formed by the GCV. Thick epicardial adipose tissue was also present in this area. The abundance of epicardial adipose tissue overlying this area may affect arrhythmogenic processes and electrophysiologic procedures within this region. Meanwhile, the inferior/accessible area has an irregular shape and is formed by the GCV/AIV and arcuate line. The density of coronary branches and epicardial adipose tissue in this area is significantly lower than that of the superior/inaccessible region,[4,11] making it more "accessible" for mapping and ablation. Because of the complexity of the spatial and anatomic relationship between LVS and surrounding epicardial structures, the epicardial approach through percutaneous pericardial puncture increases the risk of major and minor complications, such as intrapericardial bleeding, coronary artery stenosis, and delayed tamponade.[12] Therefore, the most effective and successful ablation of LVS VA is often achieved by targeting adjacent structures, such as LCC, the coronary venous system, particularly the GCV/AIV junction, or the subvalvular region of the LV endocardium. In this regard, it is important to have proper knowledge of this region to safely access, map, and ablate arrhythmias originating from the LVS.

OUTCOMES OF DIFFERENT APPROACHES TO THE CATHETER ABLATION OF LEFT VENTRICULAR SUMMIT VENTRICULAR ARRHYTHMIA
Standard Approach via Coronary Venous System and Endocardial Adjacent Structures

An increasing number of studies have indicated that catheter ablation is effective in eliminating VA originating from LVS (**Table 1** summarizes the clinical outcomes of VA originating from the LVS or adjacent structures). Enriquez and colleagues[3] describe a practical approach to the mapping and ablation of VAs from the LVS. This approach begins with an activation mapping of the coronary venous system, with particular attention given to the GCV and AIV tributaries with their septal branches. This is followed by activation mapping of the LCC, the surrounding LV endocardium and LVOT, particularly the interleaflet triangle between LCC and right coronary cusp, and the septal RVOT to identify the earliest activation sites at these adjacent structures (**Fig. 2**). The successful elimination of LVS VA can be achieved using these various structures as vantage points. In addition, a study by Lin and colleagues[13] revealed that VAs originating from the distal GCV can be distinguished from those originating from the adjacent LV endocardium based on the unique electrocardiographic (ECG) characteristics of both early and late notches in lead III (spiked helmet sign). The investigators found that this ECG characteristic is highly specific for predicting VA origin in the distal GCV.

The outcomes of catheter ablation of LVS VAs, in general, range from 22% to 100% for acute procedural success with long-term freedom from VA recurrence ranging from 23% to 100%.[4,12,14] In most approaches, catheter ablation of LVS VAs can be successfully achieved from the coronary venous system through the GCV-AIV junction (as

the earliest activation site with a good pace map of 12/12[15]) with an acute success rate of 27–74%.[5,6,8] Notably, the success rate is variable in each study and could be due to differences in the technical approach to the mapping and ablation of VA from adjacent structures, power settings used, and anatomy of the coronary venous system, such as the inability to advance the catheter to the site of interest owing to the small size of the vessel or the size and characteristics of the study population. A study by Yamada and colleagues[4] showed that the prevalence of LV summit VA origin was found within the GCV/AIV junction and could be successfully ablated from within this area in 14 of 27 (52%) of their cases, whereas the remaining was achieved through adjacent structures. In addition, a previous study by Jauregui Abularach and colleagues[16] showed that although the earliest activation site and best pace map (12/12) were in the distal GCV or proximal AIV, successful ablation was also achieved in adjacent structures, particularly LSOV in 8 out of 9 (89%) cases; these studies only included a small number of patients. However, in the most recent multicenter study by Chung and colleagues[17] that included 238 patients with LVS VA who underwent catheter ablation, the result showed acute ablation outcomes for LVS VA from different ablation sites. In 199 of these patients, 78 (39.2%) were successfully ablated at the GCV/AIV through the coronary venous system, 62 (31.2%) from the aortic sinus of Valsalva (ASV), and 40 (20.1%) from the subvalvular area. In 105 (51.8%) patients, multiple ablation sites were required to achieve acute success, suggesting possible intramural foci, or it could be due to a more complex substrate contributing to higher recurrences despite achieving acute procedural success. Multisite ablation (≥2 sites) for VA elimination was also found to predict long-term VA recurrence after an initial successful independent ablation. Furthermore, this is also the first study to report long-term freedom from LVS VA recurrence after catheter ablation. Overall, the acute success rate using standard ablation of LVS VA was 81.6%, and after a mean follow-up period of 26 months, the freedom from VA recurrence was 83.6%. The investigators found that most recurrent VAs that occurred within 1 year had a QRS morphology similar to that identified before ablation. This indicates that the main reason for failed ablation of adjacent anatomic structures and VA recurrence would be the inability to eliminate VA owing to lack of proximity to epicardial or intramural arrhythmogenic foci, inadequate ablation, or poor energy penetration, as previously reported.[18,19]

Table 1
Clinical outcomes of ventricular arrhythmias originating from the left ventricular summit or adjacent structures

Study, Year of Publication	Case Number	LVS Access	Strategy	Acute Success Rate, %	Follow-Up Period, mo	Recurrences, %	Note
Yamada et al,[1] 2016	45	GCV, AMC, LCC	Unipolar ablation	73.3	Median: 55	0	LVOT VAs with earliest activation site on the epicardial sites > earliest endocardial site by 10 milliseconds
Liao et al,[7] 2020	20 patients with VA with abrupt transition in lead V3; 6 with epicardial origin	1 at LCC and 5 at RCC/LCC interleaflet triangle	Unipolar ablation	100	Mean: 12 ± 11	11	VA with abrupt transition in lead V3; 6 with epicardial origin (4 at GCV/AIV and 2 at the proximal LAD)
Nagashima et al,[8] 2014	30	GCV, LV endocardium, LCC, epicardium	Unipolar ablation, cryoablation	53	Median: 2.8	18.8	
Chung et al,[17] 2020	238	GCV, LV endocardium, LCC, epicardium	Unipolar ablation, bipolar ablation	83.6	Median: 26	17.80	
Shirai et al,[19] 2019	65	LVOT, LCC, RCC/LCC interleaflet triangle, RVOT	Unipolar ablation	49	Median: 11.5	15	Anatomic approach
Futyma et al,[21] 2020	4	LV endocardium and GCV/AIC	Bipolar ablation	100	Mean: 15 ± 4	0	Bipolar ablation from GCV/AIV and adjacent endocardium
Futyma et al,[22] 2020	7	LCC and LVOT	Bipolar ablation	71.4 with VA suppression	Mean: 14 ± 6	NA	Mean 84% of PVC reduction

Abbreviations: NA, not applicable; PVC, premature ventricular complex.

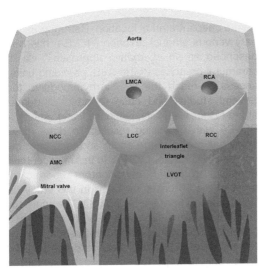

Fig. 2. The vantage area surrounding the sinuses of Valsalva and LVOT for ablation of LV summit VA. Detailed mapping of supravalvular and subvalvular area, especially for right-left aortic interleaflet triangle, may successfully ablate the LVS VA without epicardial approaches. AMC, aortomitral continuity; NCC, noncoronary cusp; RCA, right coronary artery; RCC, right coronary cusp.

Percutaneous Epicardial Approach

When the successful elimination of LVS VA could not be achieved from the coronary venous system or adjacent endocardial sites, a percutaneous epicardial approach was attempted. This can be performed using an anterior or posterior epicardial approach depending on the experience and preference of the operator, as well as the patient-specific risk assessment. Studies reporting the outcomes of LVS VA ablation using a percutaneous epicardial approach remain limited. A study by Santangeli and colleagues[20] included 23 consecutive patients with LVS VA who had previously unsuccessful ablation of LVS VA from the coronary venous system and multiple LV and RV endocardial sites and underwent percutaneous epicardial ablation. RF ablation of the epicardium was attempted in 14 patients (61%). Five (22%) patients achieved acute elimination of VA, and they found that in all 5 successful ablations, the origins of the VAs were localized at the most lateral basal part of the LVS triangle or the "accessible area" of the LVS. In contrast, 9 (39%) patients did not achieve acute success and could probably be due to the presence of epicardial fat that inhibits adequate energy delivery to the epicardium. RF energy delivery was not attempted in 9 (39%) patients owing to proximity to the LAD or LCx arteries. Overall, in this series of 23 patients, the

ablation outcomes were poor, with an acute success rate of 22%, and the long-term freedom from VA recurrence was 17%. Similarly, in the study by Yamada and colleagues,[4] 9 out of 27 (33%) patients underwent percutaneous epicardial ablation, but only 4 (44%) of these patients were successfully ablated. The successful site of ablation in these patients was achieved on the epicardial surface lateral and inferior to the GCV/AIV (accessible area). In 4 other patients, epicardial mapping revealed the earliest ventricular activation at the apex of the LVS triangle, which was bounded by the LAD and LCx and superior to the GCV/AIV (inaccessible area). Pacing from endocardial or epicardial sites surrounding LVS in these 4 patients cannot yield an excellent pace map. Therefore, attempts to deliver RF energy were abandoned owing to their proximity to the coronary arteries. However, in this study, long-term freedom from VA recurrence was not reported. A multicenter collaborative study by Chung and colleagues[17] was the first to demonstrate overall long-term freedom from VA recurrence in patients with LVS VA who underwent ablation but did not specifically mention the long-term success rate of the percutaneous epicardial approach because of the limited number of cases using this particular approach. In 97 of the 238 (40.7%) patients who underwent initial ablation targeting the epicardial area, 91 (93.8%) were via the coronary venous system, and 6 (6.2%) were via a percutaneous epicardial approach. Successful elimination of VA was achieved by epicardial ablation in 40 (41.2%) patients. Among these, only 3 of the 6 patients who initially underwent the percutaneous epicardial approach achieved acute success. In those with a failed first approach to ASV, successful elimination was achieved using the second approach when targeting VA using the percutaneous epicardial approach. The investigators also reported that targeting the LVS area through epicardial access was not associated with better acute procedural success than the initial approach to an endocardial structure. The acute success rate of the percutaneous epicardial approach in this study was 9.5%. Overall, the success rates for ablation of LVS VA from the epicardium remained low, even in the accessible region. Possible reasons for the failure of the epicardial approach to eliminate VA were similar to those reported in previous studies.[4,21]

Bipolar Radiofrequency Catheter Ablation

Bipolar radiofrequency catheter ablation (RFCA) is an emerging option for arrhythmias that are less accessible, or when ablation with conventional unipolar energy sources may be challenging or impossible. To date, a few studies have reported their experience with bipolar ablation of the LVS VA. Futyma and colleagues[21] reported 4 highly symptomatic patients who underwent bipolar ablation for recurrent LVS VA with previous unipolar RFCA at the earliest site in GCV/AIV and the second best location in the LVOT and aortic cusp. In 2 patients, a late recurrence of the clinical ventricular premature complex (VPC) was observed, whereas in the other 2 patients, previous unipolar ablation did not cause any suppression of VA. Acute success was achieved in all patients through bipolar ablation at the earliest site of activation in the GCV/AIV and opposite endocardium. In two of these patients, bipolar ablation was performed safely using repetitive angiography of the LMCA and its branches during ablation. At follow-up, all patients remained asymptomatic without VT recurrence and with a decrease in VPC burden of a mean of 83%. Cardiac MRI also demonstrated transmural lesions after bipolar ablation. In this study, the investigators demonstrated the safe and effective delivery of bipolar RF energy to the GCV/AVI and opposite endocardium. However, this approach requires optimal anatomy and may not always be applicable for LVS VA, especially those originating from inaccessible areas. Futyma and colleagues[22] demonstrated an effective and alternative approach using bipolar RF delivery to the LPC and opposite LVOT in patients with VA originating from the inaccessible area of the LVS. In a series of 7 patients, acute success was achieved in 5 (71%) patients. In two of the cases, bipolar ablation was performed successfully using dextrose 5% in water to improve lesion formation. After a mean follow-up of 14 ± 6 months, there was no recurrence of VT in 2 patients with baseline VT and a mean 84% decrease in the burden of VPC in the other patients. Finally, the study by Igarashi and colleagues,[23] which included 18 patients with underlying structural heart disease, demonstrated a successful acute suppression of VA in 5 patients with LVS VA without complications. In a 12-month follow-up period, 3 patients were free from VA recurrence, 1 patient had VA recurrence in the fifth month postablation and was maintained on medication thereafter, and 1 patient died of heart failure in the fifth month postablation.

Retrograde Coronary Venous Ethanol Ablation

RF catheter ablation of LVS VA via the endocardial or epicardial approach may fail owing to inaccessibility of the substrate, that is, the origin may be located in the inaccessible region of the LVS or from a deep intramural location. Retrograde coronary venous ethanol ablation (RCVEA) has been described as an alternative approach[24] via the intramural branches of the CVS, providing unique access to reach the LVS arrhythmogenic foci. Several studies and case reports[24–29] demonstrated the feasibility, efficacy, and safety of RCVEA with promising results. To date, only 1 study has reported the acute and long-term outcomes of RCVEA for LVS VA. In this multicenter international registry,[28] investigators reported that most of the 56 cases included in this study had VA originating from the LVS (76%). The acute success for VA elimination with RCVEA was 55 of 56 patients (98%) with a long-term freedom from VA recurrence of 77% after 1 year of follow-up. There were only 2 reported complications, that is, venous dissections from venous instrumentation leading to pericardial effusion, but none were directly secondary to ethanol infusion.

SUMMARY

The ablation of LVS VA remains challenging, and the acute success rate is far from uniform, particularly owing to the difficulties in reaching the VT substrate and differences in the technical approach to mapping and ablation. In most approaches, catheter ablation of LVS VAs can be achieved successfully from adjacent endocardial sites or the coronary venous system through the GCV-AIV junction with long-term freedom from VA recurrence of 86%. When this is unsuccessful, a percutaneous epicardial approach may be attempted or other alternative strategies, such as bipolar ablation from 2 adjacent anatomic sites or RCVEA, may be used to achieve acute success. However, because of the scarcity of available studies, additional investigations with a larger cohort of patients are warranted to clearly demonstrate the long-term efficacy of these alternative strategies.

CLINICS CARE POINTS

- The complex spatial anatomic relationship between the left ventricular summit and the adjacent structure poses a serious challenge to radiofrequency catheter ablation of ventricular arrhythmia originating in this region. Anatomic conditions, such as the presence of thick myocardium, epicardial fat, proximity of coronary vessels, and accessibility of the substrate, play a significant role in effective lesion formation during ablation.

- A comprehensive stepwise approach for mapping and ablation of ventricular arrhythmias from the left ventricular summit using various adjacent structures as vantage points should be performed, as catheter ablation of left ventricular summit ventricular arrhythmias can be successfully achieved from the coronary venous system and endocardial adjacent sites.

- Acute elimination of left ventricular summit ventricular arrhythmia using a percutaneous epicardial approach can be considered in patients with ventricular arrhythmia arising from the most lateral basal part of the left ventricular summit triangle or the "accessible area" of the left ventricular summit. The most common reason for failed ablation attempts with this approach was the location of the ventricular arrhythmia origin close to the coronary vessels.

- Bipolar radiofrequency catheter ablation and retrograde coronary venous ethanol ablation are 2 alternative strategies that can be performed safely to achieve acute success for the ablation of left ventricular summit ventricular arrhythmia when the standard approach or percutaneous epicardial approach is unsuccessful.

ACKNOWLEDGMENTS

This work was supported by the Ministry of Science and Technology (MOST 109-2314-B-075-075-MY3, MOST 109-2314-B-010-058-MY2, MOST 109-2314-B-075-074-MY3, MOST 109-2314-B-075 -076 -MY3, MOST 107-2314-B-010-061-MY2, MOST 106-2314-B-075-006-MY3, MOST 106-2314-B-010-046-MY3, and MOST 106-2314-B-075-073-MY3), Research Foundation of Cardiovascular Medicine, Szu-Yuan Research Foundation of Internal Medicine, Taiwan and Taipei Veterans General Hospital, Taiwan (grant numbers V106C-158, V106C-104, V107C-060, V107C-054, V108C-107, V109C-113, and V110C-116).

DISCLOSURE

F.P. Chung: Speaker honorarium from Abbott Medical, Biosense Webster, and Boston Scientific.

REFERENCES

1. Yamada T, Doppalapudi H, Litovsky SH, et al. Challenging radiofrequency catheter ablation of idiopathic ventricular arrhythmias originating from the left ventricular summit near the left main coronary artery. Circ Arrhythm Electrophysiol 2016;9(10): e004202.

2. Letsas KP, Efremidis M, Vlachos K, et al. Catheter ablation of ventricular arrhythmias arising from the distal great cardiac vein. Heart Lung Circ 2016;25: e37–40.

3. Enriquez A, Malavassi F, Saenz LC, et al. How to map and ablate left ventricular summit arrhythmias. Heart Rhythm 2017;14(1):141–8.

4. Yamada T, McElderry HT, Doppalapudi H, et al. Idiopathic ventricular arrhythmias originating from the left ventricular summit: anatomic concepts relevant to ablation. Circ Arrhythm Electrophysiol 2010;3(6):616–23.

5. Baman TS, Ilg KJ, Gupta SK, et al. Mapping and ablation of epicardial idiopathic ventricular arrhythmias from within the coronary venous system. Circ Arrhythm Electrophysiol 2010;3(3):274–9.

6. Daniels DV, Lu YY, Morton JB, et al. Idiopathic epicardial left ventricular tachycardia originating remote from the sinus of Valsalva: electrophysiological characteristics, catheter ablation, and identification from the 12-lead electrocardiogram. Circulation 2006;113(13):1659–66.

7. Liao HT, Wei W, Tanaga KS, et al. Left ventricular summit arrhythmias with an abrupt V3 transition: anatomy of the aortic interleaflet triangle vantage point. Heart Rhythm 2021;18(1):10–9.

8. Nagashima K, Choi EK, Lin KY, et al. Ventricular arrhythmias near the distal great cardiac vein: challenging arrhythmia for ablation. Circ Arrhythm Electrophysiol 2014;7:906–12.

9. McAlpine WA. Heart and coronary arteries. New York (NY): Springer-Verlag; 1975.

10. Kuniewicz M, Krupinski M, Gosnell M, et al. Applicability of computed tomography preoperative assessment of the left atrial appendage in left ventricular summit ablations. J Interv Card Electrophysiol 2021;61(2):357–63.

11. Kuniewicz M, Baszko A, Ali D, et al. Left Ventricular Summit - concept, anatomical structure and clinical significance. Diagnostics 2021;11(8):1423.

12. Lin CY, Chung FP, Lin YJ, et al. Radiofrequency catheter ablation of ventricular arrhythmias originating from the continuum between the aortic sinus of Valsalva and the left ventricular summit: electrocardiographic characteristics and correlative anatomy. Heart Rhythm 2016;13:111–21.

13. Lin YN, Xu J, Pan YQ, et al. An electrocardiographic sign of idiopathic ventricular tachycardia ablatable from the distal great cardiac vein. Heart Rhythm 2020;17:905–14.

14. Chen YH, Lin JF. Catheter ablation of idiopathic epicardial ventricular arrhythmias originating from the vicinity of the coronary sinus system. J Cardiovasc Electrophysiol 2015;26:1160–7.

15. Kodali S, Santangeli P. Mapping and ablation of arrhythmias from uncommon sites (aortic cusp,

pulmonary artery, and left ventricular summit). Card Electrophysiol Clin 2019;11:665–74.

16. Jauregui Abularach ME, Campos B, Park KM, et al. Ablation of ventricular arrhythmias arising near the anterior epicardial veins from the left sinus of Valsalva region: ECG features, anatomic distance, and outcome. Heart Rhythm 2012;9:865–73.

17. Chung FP, Lin CY, Shirai Y, et al. Outcomes of catheter ablation of ventricular arrhythmias originating from the left ventricular summit: a multicenter study. Heart rhythm 2020;17(7):1077–83.

18. Muser D, Santangeli P. Ventricular arrhythmias linked to the left ventricular summit communicating veins: a new mapping approach for an old ablation problem. Circ Arrhythm Electrophysiol 2018;11: e006105.

19. Shirai Y, Santangeli P, Liang JJ, et al. Anatomical proximity dictates successful ablation from adjacent sites for outflow tract ventricular arrhythmias linked to the coronary venous system. Europace 2019;21: 484–91.

20. Santangeli P, Lin D, Marchlinski FE. Catheter ablation of ventricular arrhythmias arising from the left ventricular summit. Card Electrophysiol Clin 2016; 8:99–107.

21. Futyma P, Sander J, Ciapala K, et al. Bipolar radiofrequency ablation delivered from coronary veins and adjacent endocardium for treatment of refractory left ventricular summit arrhythmias. J Interv Card Electrophysiol 2020;58(3):307–13.

22. Futyma P, Santangeli P, Purerfellner H, et al. Anatomic approach with bipolar ablation between the left pulmonic cusp and left ventricular outflow tract for left ventricular summit arrhythmias. Heart Rhythm 2020;17:1519–27.

23. Igarashi M, Nogami A, Fukamizu S, et al. Acute and long-term results of bipolar radiofrequency catheter ablation of refractory ventricular arrhythmias of deep intramural origin. Heart Rhythm 2020;17:1500–7.

24. Okishige K, Nakamura R, Yamauchi Y, et al. Chemical ablation of ventricular tachycardia arising from the left ventricular summit. Clin Case Rep 2019; 7(11):2036–41.

25. Sasaki T, Yamashita S, Suzuki M, et al. Successful ablation with ethanol infusion to coronary sinus branch in a case with scar-related ventricular tachycardia with left ventricular epicardial reentrant circuit. Heart Rhythm Case Rep 2020;6(4):226–9.

26. Baszko A, Kalmucki P, Siminiak T, et al. Telescopic coronary sinus cannulation for mapping and ethanol ablation of arrhythmia originating from left ventricular summit. Cardiol J 2020;27(3):312–5.

27. Kato K, Tanaka A, Hasegawa S, et al. Successful ethanol injection into the anterior interventricular cardiac vein for ventricular premature contractions arising from the left ventricular summit. Heart Rhythm Case Rep 2018;4(7):310–3.

28. Tavares L, Lador A, Fuentes S, et al. Intramural venous ethanol infusion for refractory ventricular arrhythmias: outcomes of a multicenter experience, prospective international registry. JACC Clin Electrophysiol 2020;6(11):1420–31. https://doi.org/10.1016/j.jacep.2020.07.023.

29. Baher A, Shah DJ, Valderrábano M. Coronary venous ethanol infusion for the treatment of refractory ventricular tachycardia. Heart Rhythm 2012; 9(10):1637–9.

Preventing Complications During Mapping and Ablation of Left Ventricular Summit Arrhythmias

Alejandro Jimenez Restrepo, MD, FRACP, FHRS[a,b,*],
Luis Carlos Saenz Morales, MD, FHRS[c,d]

KEYWORDS

• Ablation • Radiofrequency • Intramural • Epicardial • Ethanol injection • Bipolar • Injury

KEY POINTS

- Detailed discussion of reported complications related to left ventricular (LV) summit ventricular arrhythmia (VA) ablations.
- Understand the intricate relationship of critical structures within the LV summit and its boundaries and the risk of collateral injury related to catheter proximity, energy source, and delivery technique.
- Propose an individualized approach to LV summit ablations that includes imaging modalities such as coronary angiogram, intracardiac echocardiography, and computed tomography/MRI fusion with 3-dimensional maps to assess proximity of critical structures and prevent complications or to promptly recognize them and institute immediate action and avoid potentially fatal outcomes.

 Video content accompanies this article at http://www.cardiacep.theclinics.com.

INTRODUCTION

The left ventricular (LV) summit is a well-known site of origin (SOO) for idiopathic ventricular arrhythmias (VAs).[1] With advancements in mapping techniques and introduction of different energy sources,[2–11] SOO considered inaccessible to the electrophysiologist in the past can now be approached without the need for open thoracic access.[12,13] Nonetheless, the LV summit remains a complex anatomical region where critical structures reside or remain in its close proximity and are therefore liable to injury during ablation. In order to safely and effectively diagnose and treat these arrhythmias in the cardiac electrophysiology laboratory, it is critical to have an anatomical understanding of the 3-dimensional (3D) landmarks of this space.[14–18]

In this article, the authors review relevant known complications related to ablation of ventricular arrhythmias arising from the LV summit and its vicinity, present the unique advantages and disadvantages of each ablation technique, and discuss the role of an individualized anatomical approach to reduce procedural related complications and improve outcomes.

ANATOMICAL CONSIDERATIONS

The LV summit is a triangular space located in the superior-most aspect of the LV ostium. The bifurcation of the left main coronary artery (LMCA) defines its superior apex. Its borders are defined by a

a Marshfield Clinic Health System, 1000 North Oak Avenue, Marshfield, WI 54449, USA; b University of Maryland School of Medicine, Baltimore, MD, USA; c International Arrhythmia Center, Fundacion CardioInfantil, Bogota, Colombia; d Fundacion CardioInfantil, Instituto de Cardiologia, Calle 163 #13b-60, Bogota, Colombia
* Corresponding author.
E-mail address: Jimenezrestrepo.alejandro@marshfieldclinic.org

Card Electrophysiol Clin 15 (2023) 93–109
https://doi.org/10.1016/j.ccep.2022.07.004
1877-9182/23/© 2022 Elsevier Inc. All rights reserved.

mitral or lateral margin, close to the left circumflex artery (LCX) and a septal or medial margin close to the left anterior descending artery (LAD). Its base (most inferior portion) is delineated by an imaginary curved line with its radius determined by the distance from the left coronary artery bifurcation to the first septal perforator branch. The anterior interventricular vein (AIV) becomes the grater cardiac vein (GCV) as it enters the posterior aspect of the atrioventricular (AV) groove[14,18] and divides the LV summit into 2 areas: one superior or basal, known as the *inaccessible area*, due to its proximity to the coronary arteries and the risk of injury with catheter ablation, and one inferior or apical, known as the *accessible area,* where ablation therapy is generally considered safe and usually approachable via the GCV/AIV or its communicating veins.[19] Relevant structures near the apex of the LV summit include the aortic root and the aortoventricular membrane. Deeper structures include the left coronary cusp (LCC) at its apical margin, right coronary cusp (RCC) at its septal margin, and aortomitral continuity (AMC) at its mitral margin. The pulmonary trunk and pulmonary annulus are located above the LV summit at the most superior portion of the septal margin, whereas the right ventricular outflow tract (RVOT) overlies the inferior portion of the septal margin. Finally, The LCX and the left lateral cardiac nerve overlie the mitral margin, close to the mitral annulus (most inferior portion of the LV summit) where a small portion of the GCV is also present. Anatomical variants within the LV summit are present in up to 10% of hearts, and therefore, an individualized approach must be considered for each patient.[18] Knowledge of the spatial relationship between the LV summit and its adjacent structures (**Fig. 1**, Video 1) provides the anatomical understanding to identify potential locations where arrhythmias can be safely mapped and ablated in this area.

COMPLICATIONS

Although reported complications of LV summit VA ablations are rare, their true incidence may be underestimated due to underreporting of identified cases and misdiagnosis of cases with late complications or out-of-hospital fatal outcome. In the largest multicentric registry of LV summit VA published to date, Chung and colleagues[20] evaluated procedural related outcomes of 238 patients from 4 international centers. A total of 7 procedural related complications were reported (**Table 1**). There were no procedural related deaths during a mean follow-up period of 25 ± 20 months. Individual case reports and case series of

complications related to ablation of VAs arising from or near the LV summit region are analyzed below and summarized in **Table 1**. These complications can be grouped by energy source utilized and delivery method.

Unipolar Radiofrequency– and Cryoenergy Ablation–Related Complications

Two case reports of LV pseudoaneurysm occurring after LV summit ablation are reported in the literature. Dandamudi and colleagues[21] reported a late presenting and recurrent hemopericardium and cardiac tamponade in a 52-year-old woman, occurring 3 and 8 weeks following a combined atrial fibrillation ablation and premature ventricular contraction (PVCs) ablation approached from the LCC and the LV endocardium below the cusp using irrigated radiofrequency (RF) ablation. The recurrent hemopericardium was initially thought to represent a severe form of Dressler syndrome. A cardiac MRI following the second admission confirmed the diagnosis of a pseudoaneurysm in the basal anterior LV below the aortic valve. A total of 240 seconds of RF ablation between 30 and 50 Watts (W) were delivered at the LV endocardial site during the procedure, with a maximal impedance drop of 29 Ω and an average contact force between 22 and 26 grams. In retrospect, the initial postprocedural computed tomography (CT) scan had shown a large LV pseudoaneurysm but was misinterpreted as an enlarged left atrial appendage. The patient underwent successful surgical exclusion of the pseudoaneurysm with a bovine pericardial patch. The authors hypothesize that a combination of high-power energy and long duration of the ablation lesions likely contributed to this complication. Darma and colleagues[22] reported the case of a 25-year-old man with highly symptomatic frequent PVCs arising from the LV. Endocardial mapping localized earliest signals to the anterolateral aspect of the mitral annulus (MA). Epicardial mapping from the distal coronary sinus (CS) showed earliest activation at the distal GCV. Initial endocardial ablation was performed with an irrigated tip catheter (50 W, maximum temperature of 42°C) followed by epicardial ablation at the earliest GCV site (20 to 25 W, frequently interrupted due to steep impedance drops) and only achieving transient PVC suppression. Percutaneous epicardial access was eventually required, with earliest epicardial activation confirmed in the region of the LV summit. Following coronary angiogram, an extensive ablation was performed (40 to 45 W, irrigated catheter) until the PVCs were eliminated acutely (unknown total ablation time, no steam pops or significant impedance

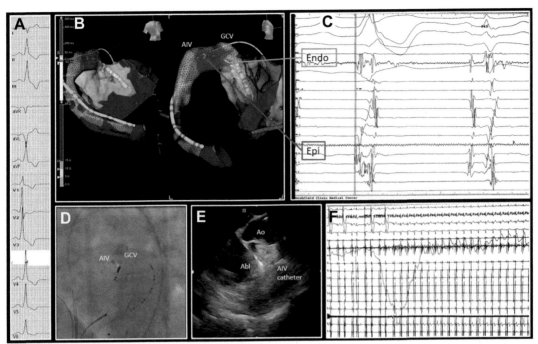

Fig. 1. A 65-year-old woman with PVCs (ectopic burden 27%) and NSVT arising from the LVOT. Twelve-lead ECG showing an RBBB morphology, inferior axis, and positive precordial concordance with a slurred QRS upstroke (A). Three-dimensional electroanatomical mapping from the infravlvular LVOT (endocardium) using a 4-mm irrigated catheter and the GCV/AIV junction using a 3 F multielectrode catheter confirmed earliest ventricular activation in the LV summit region (B). Epicardial local activation was −32 ms preQRS (red arrow) and 6 ms before endocardial activation (orange arrow) (C). Ablation from the endocardial LVOT under the aortic valve (orange arrowhead) and opposite the GCV/AIV earliest activation site (red arrowhead) is seen on fluoroscopy (D) and ICE (E), in a safe area away from coronary arteries. Immediate PVC suppression was observed with RF ablation at 30 W (F). This figure highlights the importance of complimentary imaging modalities to understand the 3D spatial landmarks of the LV summit and adjacent structures to guide the ablation approach. Abl, ablation catheter; Ao, aortic valve.

drops reported). Transthoracic echocardiogram (TTE) postoperatively showed no pericardial effusion. Three weeks postprocedure, the patient was readmitted with angina, dyspnea, and syncope. Electrocardiogram (ECG) showed ST segment elevation in inferolateral leads. TTE confirmed a large pericardial effusion with tamponade, a pseudoaneurysm in the lateral LV wall, and a defect in the mitral valve. Patient underwent pericardiocentesis, and a coronary angiogram excluded coronary artery lesions. Emergency open heart surgery was performed (pericardial patch to close a defect underneath the aortic valve between the LCC and the A1 segment of the mitral valve plus mitral valve repair). Postoperative cardiac MRI showed a persistent small defect in the LV region previously repaired, initially managed conservatively. Three months later, a second surgery was required (pericardial patch aortic reconstruction). Eventually the patient recovered without further evidence of pseudoaneurysm

formation, leaks, or hemodynamic complications. The authors postulate an inaudible steam pop as a possible cause of this complication.

The mechanism of an LV pseudoaneurysm formation after catheter ablation for ventricular tachycardias (VTs) or PVCs from the LV summit relates to a myocardial perforation secondary to tissue necrosis from thermal injury (from steam pops or large volume thermal lesions) that is contained by a thin tissue layer, thus preventing acute hemodynamic deterioration, but with risk of later developing intermittent leakage, causing late presenting cardiac tamponade (as occurred in both these cases), or frank rupture, leading to sudden cardiac death. Both these cases share common characteristics: Normal structural hearts, RF energy used, and extended applications with high power and multisite applications. An important impedance drop was not associated with a visual steam pop in the first case (intracardiac echocardiography [ICE] was used), and no

Table 1
Reported LV summit complications

Reference	Complication	Energy Source	Technique	Approach	Outcome	Observations
Dandamudi et al,[21] 2017	LV pseudoaneurysm	Irrigated RF	Unipolar	LCC, LV endo	Pericardiocenthesis, surgical repair	Combined with AF ablation. High-power RF. Late presenting tamponade. DX confirmed by CMR.
Darma et al,[22] 2021	LV pseudoaneurysm	Irrigated RF	Unipolar	LV endo, GCV/AV, V Epi	Pericardiocenthesis, surgical repair X2	High-power RF, MV repair, and LV pseudoaneurysm and Ao reconstruction.
Nakatani et al,[26] 2021	Coronary injury	Irrigated RF	Unipolar	Septal RVOT	PCI	Mid-LAD occlusion requiring PCI with thrombus aspiration. 35 W and high contact force (>50 gm intermittently).
Benhayon et al,[27] 2017	Coronary injury	Irrigated RF	Unipolar	Anteroseptal RVOT	PCI	Abl at the RV anterior horn. 40 W/ 60 sec.
Pons et al,[30] 1997	Coronary injury	RF	Unipolar	LV endo	No intervention	Chronic LMCA occlusion (w/ collaterals) 2 years post-RF ablation. No RF ablation details of exact location or RF parameters.
Steven et al,[31] 2013	Coronary injury (N = 1)	Irrigated RF	Unipolar	LV endo, GCV/Av	PCI	LCX occlusion, RF site was 2 mm from coronary, avg 23 W.
	Coronary injury (N = 1)	Irrigated RF	Unipolar	LV endo, GCV/Av	PCI	LCX occlusion, RF site was 5–7 mm from coronary, avg 27W.
	GCV perforation (N = 1)	Irrigated RF	Unipolar	LV endo, GCV/Av	No intervention	During catheter instrumentation, no tamponade.
	Coronary spasm (N = 1)	Cryoablation	Surgical	LV Epi	PCI	Intraprocedural LAD spasm and acute LV dysfunction. Focal LAD lesion during FUP
Kordic et al,[33] 2018	Coronary dissection	NA	NA	LV endo	PCI	LAD dissection during retrograde Ao catheter advancement.

Study	Complication				Outcome	Comments
Keegan et al,[34] 2021	Aortic dissection	NA	NA	LV endo	Death	Source likely iliac dissection during sheath exchange. Predisposing aortopathy? Acute type A aortic dissection with hemopericardium, flap seen on ICE and CT. Emergency surgical repair. Died of post-op complications.
Kumar et al,[10] 2015	Coronary vasospasm	Ethanol	TCEA	Intracoronary	No intervention	Not specified if LVOT case or non-LVOT case (part of a case series).
Tavares et al,[11] 2020	Cardiac tamponade (N = 2)	Ethanol	Intramural venous	GCV/AIV	Pericardiocentesis	Due to venous instrumentation.
	Cardiac tamponade (N = 1)	RF (wire)	Intramural venous	GCV/AIV	Pericardiocentesis	Due to vessel perforation during wire ablation using an electrocautery pen.
	Pericarditis (N = 1)	Ethanol	Intramural venous	GCV/AIV	Oral Colchicine	Suspected to be related to ethanol infusion.
Stevenson et al,[38] 2019	Intramyocardial bleb (N = 1)	Needle RF	Intramural	LV intramural endo	Pericardiocentesis	Observed on ICE, lead to small pericardial effusion (110 m) without tamponade, drained for safety concerns.
Nguyen et al,[5] 2018	Steam pops (N = 12)	Irrigated RF	Unipolar + HNS	LV endo/LV epi	No intervention	LV summit cases included but aso from other area (not specified). No perforations related to steam pops.
Chung et al,[20] 2020	Cardiac tamponade (N = 2)	RF	Unipolar	LV endo, GCV/AIV, LV, Epi, ASV	Pericardiocentesis	During mapping of distal CS.
	CS dissection (N = 1)	RF	Unipolar	LV endo, GCV/AIV, LV, Epi, ASV	No Intervention	Asymptomatic, no tamponade
	Coronary spasm (N = 1)	RF	Unipolar	LV endo, GCV/AIV, LV, Epi, ASV	No intervention	Transient
	Coronary injury (N = 1)	RF	Unipolar	LV endo, GCV/AIV, LV, Epi, ASV	NA	Symptomatic, late presenting during FUP

1. From Kumar et al,[10] subgroup-related complications were not specified.
2. No complications reported from bipolar RF targeting LV summit substrates in several case series.[12,13,42]
3. Data from Chung et al[20] does not specify type of RF ablation (irrigated vs nonirrigated) or approach (endocardial vs epicardial) for each complication.

obvious impedance changes or audible pops were seen during ablation in the second case (no ICE was used). High-energy RF applications over extended periods of time in a small circumscribed area (consolidation lesions) or adjacent areas equidistant to an intramural SOO (sequential ablations) may predispose to this complication. An inaudible steam pop may have led to gas formation and rupture. Although a significant impedance drop during extensive RF ablation should prompt the operator to terminate RF application, as this may precede a steam pop, it is not a prerequisite for tissue gas formation.[23] Although the LV is regarded as being highly resistant to perforation during catheter ablation procedures owing to its wall thickness, tamponade and perforation during RF ablation of scar-mediated VTs in areas of ventricular wall thinning has been reported.[24] Unlike RF ablations performed above the aortic valve (at the cusp or commissural plane) where the RF energy has to penetrate fibrous aortic wall, leaflet tissue, and epicardial fat to reach the adjacent myocardium; ablations below the aortic cusps, at the right-to-left aortic interleaflet triangle, result in direct contact with the myocardium of the anterior aspect of the LV ostium, where its tip culminates into an apex with a thickness less than or equal to 5 mm[25] and is therefore vulnerable to perforation during extensive RF ablation.

Nakatani and colleagues reported a case of LAD artery thermal injury following ablation of VTs originating in the right ventricular (RV) outflow tract in a 79-year-old man with dilated cardiomyopathy and recurrent syncope. A preprocedural echocardiogram showed a LV ejection fraction of 45%. A cardiac MRI showed nonspecific fibrosis in the LV posterior wall with no apparent RV abnormalities. Preprocedure coronary angiogram showed no significant coronary artery disease. A VT originating from the septal region of the RV outflow tract was mapped and ablated (irrigated tip catheter, 35 W, contact force > 50 g intermittently). No steam pops were observed and maximal impedance drop was 18 Ω. The VT was suppressed after 180 seconds of ablation; however, 2 other VTs were seen, originating from septal adjacent sites. These VTs were targeted, but after 4 minutes of RF delivery, ST elevation in the precordial leads and aVL was noted. Coronary angiogram confirmed a total occlusion of the mid-LAD. Emergency coronary angioplasty with thrombus aspiration was required. Following angioplasty, all VTs resolved. Merged 3D CT images with the electroanatomical map revealed the ablation sites were in close proximity to the midportion of the LAD epicardially. The ablation sites were 5 mm below the pulmonic valve, and the RV wall thickness at this location was 3.8 mm. Patient had no recurrent VTs at 6-month follow-up.[26] The authors postulate the thin RV myocardium and high-power RF delivery over extensive periods of time, together with high contact force values, likely led to this complication (Fig. 2). Benhayon and colleagues[27] reported the case of a 36-year-old woman with no structural heart disease (normal TTE and cardiac MRI) and exercise triggered sustained VT with a left bundle branch morphology, inferior axis, and late precordial transition. Earliest 3D activation map of her VT was localized to the RV free wall, and after an initial ablation, a similar PVC was mapped to the junction of the septum and the free wall of the RVOT, 3 cm under the pulmonic valve. RF energy delivered in this area (40 W, 60 seconds) eliminated the VT but was followed by acute chest pain with ST segment elevation in V1 to V5. Coronary angiogram confirmed an acute occlusion of the mid-LAD requiring emergent percutaneous coronary angioplasty. Patient recovered well with no recurrence of VAs and normalized LV function. Learning from this case, the authors then describe a second case of a 20-year-old man with arrhythmogenic right ventricular dysplasia who presented for ablation of RV outflow tract VTs. The authors instituted a modified approach using intracardiac echocardiography and 3D reconstruction of the LAD based on ICE images (CartoSound, Biosense Webster, CA, USA) to guide RF energy application in the septal region of the RVOT. The authors recognized the close proximity of the RVOT horn area (also referred to at RVOT site 6)[28] to the epicardial aspect of LV and the mid-LAD trajectory. The contact force vector of the ablation catheter was deviated from the LAD path by pointing the tip in an anterior (rightward) as opposed to septal (leftward) direction in order to avoid coronary injury. A very important conclusion suggested by the authors is that if RF delivery is required at the RVOT horn site (which projects toward the septum), one must reduce power and duration of ablation (no more than 20 W, 30 seconds, and 20 g of contact force). The authors also recognize that individual anatomical variations may predispose some patients to coronary injury but advocate for ICE or coronary angiogram to visualize the LAD when ablating VAs arising from this region of the RVOT.

These 2 cases highlight LAD injuries related to endocardial ablations from RV adjacent sites to the LV summit, in proximity to the LAD course in the anterior wall. Dong and colleagues described the relevant anatomical relationships between the coronary arteries, the aortic sinuses of Valsalva (ASV), the pulmonary sinuses of Valsalva (PSV), and the RVOT, after reviewing coronary CT studies

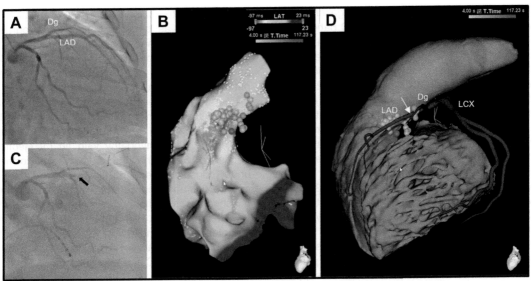

Fig. 2. Ablation in the septal RV outflow tract in a 79-year-old man with dilated cardiomyopathy and VT. (*A*) Coronary angiogram preprocedure. (*B*) 3D map anatomy and activation map of the septal aspect RV outflow tract (left posterior oblique view), with ablation lesion tags. (*C*) Intraprocedural coronary angiogram confirming acute occlusion of the mid-LAD, beyond the first diagonal branch (Dg) ostium (*black arrow*). (*D*) Reconstructed cardiac CT displaying ventricular anatomy and left coronary artery, co-registered with ablation tags from the 3D map. The region of the LAD occlusion seen on (*C*) corresponds to the white arrow, in close proximity to the ablation lesions. (*Adapted from* Nakatani Y, Vlachos K, Ramirez FD, et al. Acute coronary artery occlusion and ischemia-related ventricular tachycardia during catheter ablation in the right ventricular outflow tract. J Cardiovasc Electrophysiol. 2021;32(2):547-550. https://doi.org/10.1111/jce.14809, with permission.)

of 145 patients. Septal regions of the RVOT, particularly near the pulmonary valve, are in close proximity to the LMCA. The authors label the 3 PSV as left adjacent, right adjacent, and anterior sinuses, corresponding to the left, right, and anterior pulmonary valve cusps, respectively (LPC, RPC, and APC). The minimal distance from the LPC to the LMCA was 5.08 ± 3.9 mm and to the LAD was 3.06 ± 1.5 mm. The LMCA and LAD resided within 2 mm of the LPC in 19% and 36% of cases, respectively. Three types of anatomical relationships between the pulmonary and aortic sinuses of Valsalva were described: type 1 (intimate contact between left pulmonary and LCCs <2 mm), type 2 (close contact between the left pulmonary and LCCs, but separated by a portion of the LMCA, 2–5 mm), and type 3 (left pulmonary cusp close to the RCC and distant from the LCC, >5 mm). Prevalence of these variants was 19%, 48%, and 33%, respectively. With regard to the APC, the minimum distance from the LMCA and LAD was 16.9 ± 5.3 mm and 4.64 ± 2.2 mm, respectively. In all but one case the APC was greater than 5 mm away from the LMCA. The APC was within 5 mm from the LAD in 68% of cases and within 2 mm in 17%. The right coronary artery (RCA) is located within 5 mm of the RPC/RVOT in 82% of cases. In most cases the

closest site to the RPC/RVOT is the proximal RCA, and the mid-RCA in only 22%. Finally, the minimum distance from the pulmonary trunk (PT) to the LMCA was 4.12 ± 2.3 mm and to the LAD was 5.83 ± 3.2 mm, and in almost all cases the closest site was less than 10 mm above the sinotubular junction.[29] These anatomical observations justify caution when ablating VA arising from the PSV and the PT.

There are several case reports of coronary artery injury during ablation of LV outflow tract (LVOT) arrhythmias. Pons and colleagues reported a case of chronic LMCA occlusion 2 years following a seemingly uncomplicated ablation of an idiopathic VT from the LVOT. No details regarding the exact location, type of catheter used, total energy, or duration of RF delivery were provided.[30] Steven and colleagues reported complication rates of patients undergoing ablation of LV summit VA from within the GCV. All patients undergoing ablation from the GCV had earlier activation times in the GCV compared with adjacent endocardial sites; 14 out of 117 patients met criteria for LV summit (epicardial) VA origin. Ablation was not attempted due to proximity to a coronary artery (n = 3) or pre-existing significant CAD (n = 1). Coronary artery spasm was observed in 3 out of 10 cases, all resolving during follow-up angiogram. No other complications were reported.[31] Nagashima and colleagues reported outcomes of 30 patients undergoing catheter ablation for VAs with earliest activation in the GCV. Three patients were not ablated due to failure to advance the ablation catheter into the distal GCV. In 7 patients (23%) the target site in the GCV was greater than or equal to 5 mm from any coronaries, and ablation was safely performed. In 8 patients the target site was within 5 mm from a coronary artery, and ablation was performed 2 to 3 mm proximal to the more distal earliest activation site in order to avoid coronary artery injury (average power 23 W and duration 30 sec). In 4 patients cryoablation was attempted due to inadequate power delivery with RF (n = 3) or to reinforce a successful RF application (n = 1; −80°C, 4–8 minutes). Overall, successful ablation was only achieved in 5 patients, whereas 21 patients had no definitive VA suppression. Additional endocardial ablations from the AMC, LCC, and RV sites were performed in 12, 5, and 4 patients, respectively, following GCV ablation and successfully abolished VA in 4 (33%), 1 (20%), and 0 cases. Ten patients underwent epicardial mapping via percutaneous approach, but only 2 underwent catheter ablation, with one successful VA elimination. In the remaining 8 cases no ablation was performed due to catheter proximity to a coronary artery. Three major complications were reported. Two patients who underwent RF applications with an average power of 23 and 27 W, at sites 2 and 5 to 7 mm, respectively, from an obtuse marginal branch of the LCX, suffered coronary artery occlusion requiring stenting. One patient had catheter perforation of the GCV without tamponade. Finally, of 3 patients who underwent open-chest cryothermal surgical epicardial ablation, 2 had successful VA elimination, whereas one had ablation interrupted due to vasospasm of the LAD with transient LV dysfunction seen on intraoperative TEE. The patient developed angina and persistent LV dysfunction several months postprocedure. Angiogram revealed a significant LAD focal stenosis at the site of cryoablation, requiring placement of a drug-eluting stent.[32] The authors concluded that although LV summit VA ablation from the distal GCV is feasible when RF energy can be effectively delivered (5 of 7 patients in their series), significant limitations to successful ablation at this site exist, including proximity to coronary arteries and inability to advance the ablation catheter to a distal GCV site. Although cryoablation can overcome impedance rises that limit RF energy delivery in the GCV and reduce the risk of thermal injury, the size of the cryoablation catheter is a limitation to reach distal GCV sites in many cases.

Coronary artery injury during LVOT ablation is also reported as a complication of retrograde advancement of the ablation catheter from the aorta, causing mechanical trauma to the LMCA and/or LAD due to inadvertent cannulation of its ostium, leading to an intimal dissection.[33]

Keegan and colleagues reported a case of fatal aortic dissection in a 73-year-old woman with frequent PVCs from the LV summit and a noncompacted LV cardiomyopathy with an LV ejection fraction of 31%. The procedure was performed under conscious sedation. Right femoral arterial access was obtained without difficulty and a short 8 F sheath was exchanged over the wire for a long 8 F sheath (63 cm). A 4-mm irrigated tip ablation catheter was advanced without difficulty into the ascending aorta, aortic cusps, and LV. During mapping at the LCC and LVOT, a sudden pericardial effusion with tamponade developed. Following pericardiocentesis, a dissection flap in the ascending aorta was noted on ICE. An urgent CT confirmed an aortic dissection involving the brachiocephalic trunk and right carotid arteries cranially and the left iliac artery caudally (**Fig. 3**). The patient underwent emergency aortic valve resuspension, ascending aortic replacement, descending aortic grafting, and a femoro-femoral bypass. Postoperative course was protracted with refractory shock and mesenteric ischemia, leading to death within 24 hours of surgery.[34] The authors postulate an intimal dissection at the level of the iliac artery during sheath advancement as the likely cause of the aortic dissection. Although the complication was not related to the ablation technique or energy utilized, it is important to recognize the potential for vascular complications that can lead to life-threatening events during left-sided VA ablations using a retrograde aortic access,[35,36] and they recommend consideration for a transseptal approach to reach the LV in elderly patients in order to reduce the risk of vascular complications.

Complications Related to Ethanol Infusion, Needle Ablation, Wire Ablation, Bipolar Ablation, and Irrigated Ablation Using Low Ionic Solutions

Alternative energy sources to overcome risk of thermal injury near the coronary arteries have been explored by several groups. Tavares and colleagues[11] presented the outcomes of the largest case series reported (56 patients) on the use of intramural venous ethanol infusion for treatment of intramural VAs. Forty-eight patients with VA from the LV summit were included. All patients underwent endocardial mapping from the RV and LV

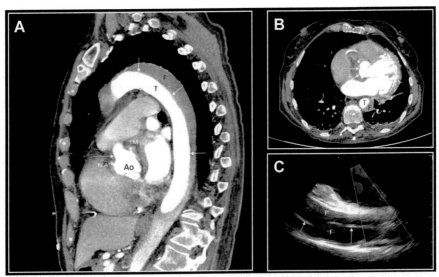

Fig. 3. Fatal aortic dissection following retrograde aortic access for LV summit PVC ablation. (*A*) shows sagittal plane of chest CT with contrast. The ascending arch and descending aorta show a double contrast density consistent with false (F) and true (T) lumens. The origin of the left main (LM) and right coronary arteries is seen. Arrows show the intimal dissection flap, which extends just above the RCA and LMCA. (*B*) A CT axial plane view at the level of the aortic annulus, showing extension of the dissection flap into the ASV. Also seen is a portion of the descending aorta, with a dissection flap separating true (T) and false (F) lumens. (*C*) Corresponding ICE images with longitudinal view of the descending aorta and a distinct intimal flap (*arrows*) separating the true (T) and false (F) lumens. (Images courtesy of Dr. Roberto Keegan.)

outflow tracts and epicardial mapping via the CS to reach the GCV/AIV region. All patients had unsuccessful RF ablation from the GCV/AIV, due to inability to either suppress VA after adequate RF delivery or to deliver adequate RF energy due to high impedances. Target branches for ethanol delivery were chosen based on earliest unipolar activation during VAs and best pace maps using a unipolar wire. Once a vein branch was chosen, the angioplasty wire was removed and contrast was injected to assess the vessel size and extent of myocardial staining. Finally, sequential 1-mL ethanol injections were delivered based on response and extent of the target area. Acute VA elimination was achieved in 38 patients (68%) using ethanol injection exclusively and in 17 patients (30%) using a combination of ethanol infusion and RF ablation near the infused vein (overall acute success 98%). At 1-year follow-up, freedom from VA was 77%. Complications included pericardial effusion in 3 patients (5%) requiring pericardiocenthesis. Two of these cases were attributed to venous instrumentation and one to RF delivery over an angioplasty wire using an electrocautery pen. One case of postprocedure pericarditis felt to be related to ethanol infusion required treatment with oral colchicine. The authors recommend this technique for ablation of LV summit arrhythmias that recur after conventional RF ablation or when

RF ablation fails to suppress the VAs using an endocardial and epicardial approach. The acute durable success seen with ethanol infusion of venous targets for VA elimination is likely due to the ability to deliver chemical ablation to intramural sites, felt to be the SOO of many idiopathic VAs in this region.[37]

Another approach to reach intramural ventricular substrates, including VAs from the LV summit, is the use of a needle catheter to deliver RF energy deep into the myocardium. Stevenson and colleagues reported their experience with an RF ablation catheter that uses an extendable/retractable 27-g needle to target intramural VA substrates in 31 patients who failed prior conventional RF ablation. The needle has a thermocouple within its lumen, can record unipolar or bipolar electrograms, and can pace from the needle tip or the catheter dome electrode. The tip of the needle is irrigated with heparinized saline during mapping (1 mL/min) and RF delivery (2 mL/min). Eighteen patients with periaortic VA were included. Overall acute procedural success was 73% for VA suppression. At 6-month follow-up, 48% of patients had freedom from VA and another 19% had a reduced VA burden. Complications included one case of pericardial fluid accumulation during LV outflow tract mapping for idiopathic VAs. The needle ablation catheter was positioned in the LV outflow tract below the aortic valve, and serial needle deployments were made to map the earliest activation site during PVCs, and needle saline injection suppressed ectopy. Conventional irrigated RF ablation at this site only suppressed PVCs transiently. Following 9 needle ablation lesions and 10 needle insertions for mapping at this site, an epicardial bleb was seen in the lateral LV on ICE (**Fig. 4**). This bleb subsequently ruptured and caused pericardial fluid accumulation without tamponade but was drained and anticoagulation was reverted. This complication was felt to be related to the infusion of saline into healthy myocardium, leading to fluid dissecting the tissue plane and creating an epicardial bleb, which then ruptured into the pericardial space. The authors compared this case with those where needle ablation was used for substrate modulation of scar-mediated VTs, where large amounts of saline can be infused via the needle catheter during mapping and ablation without any consequence. They recommend avoiding myocardial fluid injection in areas without myocardial scar during mapping and limiting irrigation only to areas targeted for ablation.[38]

Kumar and colleagues studied 67 patients with drug refractory VT with at least one failed endocardial and epicardial ablation (when indicated) to undergo transcoronary ethanol ablation (TCEA), surgical epicardial window to direct epicardial RF ablation (Epi-window), or surgical cryoablation (OR-Cryo). Fifty-two percent of patients had a VT storm in the month before the procedure, 72% of patients were receiving amiodarone, and a total of 92% were on a combination of antiarrhythmic drugs. Twelve patients from this cohort had refractory LV summit VAs and were treated as follows: 5 had suspected intramural origin close to the LV summit (3 underwent TCEA and 2 OR-Cryo), 4 had LV summit VAs in close proximity to coronaries (2 near the LAD-LCX bifurcation, 1 near a Ramus intermedius, and 1 close to a diagonal branch, all undergoing OR-Cryo), one had an LV summit VT that could not be ablated from the AIV due to inability to reach the target vessel (underwent OR-Cryo), and 2 patients with LVOT epicardial or intramural VA had OR-Cryo due to the need for concomitant open heart surgery. Procedural complications were high for TCEA (32%) and included AV block (N = 6), AV block plus stroke (N = 1), cholesterol embolization (N = 1), hypotension requiring intra-aortic balloon counterpulsation (N = 1), and coronary vasospasm (N = 1). One patient died acutely from multiorgan failure secondary to cholesterol embolization. At 30 days, 4 patients died of incessant VT and 1 from refractory heart failure. Nineteen percent of patients who underwent OR-Cryo has

complications as follows: fatal intraoperative pulmonary embolism (N = 1), mitral valve endocarditis (N = 1), transient RCA occlusion (N = 1), phrenic nerve injury (N = 1), and symptomatic LAD stenosis (N = 1). Two patients died postoperatively (endocarditis and pulmonary embolism cases). No complications were reported for the 4 patient who underwent Epi-Window. Although TCEA was effective in controlling VT storm in 70% of patients (16/23) and suppressing at least one inducible VT in 71% of cases (27/38 patients), 6- and 12-month VT recurrences were high (74% and 81%, respectively). OR-Cryo successfully terminated VT storm in 8 out of 10 patients and suppressed at least one inducible VT in 18/26 patients. VT recurrence at 6 and 12 months was 43% and 49%, respectively.[10] The authors conclude that a common cause of failure to achieve successful endocardial and/or epicardial ablation for VA is due to intramural foci or circuits, anatomical barriers to ablation, or difficulty accessing the epicardium. Because of their patient characteristics and the location of their VAs, complications and mortality were high. Case reports of successful transcoronary ethanol ablation for VAs originating in the LV anterobasal and septal regions have been published,[39,40] but caution should remain regarding this technique, as complications may arise from coronary artery instrumentation and/or ethanol injection, such as reentrant VT due to an incomplete scar homogenization, nontarget coronary artery embolization, vasospasm, and alcohol reflux into nontarget branches.[41]

Another approach to target intramural substrates is the use of *bipolar ablation* techniques, whereby RF energy is delivered between 2 catheters from 2 separate locations in order to target intramural substrates that lay in between the 2 catheter tips. Futyma and colleagues[12] presented a series of 4 patients with symptomatic PVCs whom underwent bipolar ablation after failed conventional unipolar RF ablation and antiarrhythmic drugs for VAs from the LV summit region (GCV/AIV), suboptimal mapping from adjacent endocardial sites, and at least >5 mm distance between the earliest GCV/AIV site and coronary arteries. The bipolar RF ablation setup consisted of an irrigated tip catheter acting as the RF electrode and a nonirrigated catheter connected as the return electrode (RE). Using a switchbox, the RE was connected to a second RF generator in order to collect data regarding RE tip temperature during RF ablation. Mean total bipolar RF ablation time was 244 ± 15 sec and average impedance drop was 20 to 30 Ω. Two patients experienced significant impedance rises during bipolar RF ablation

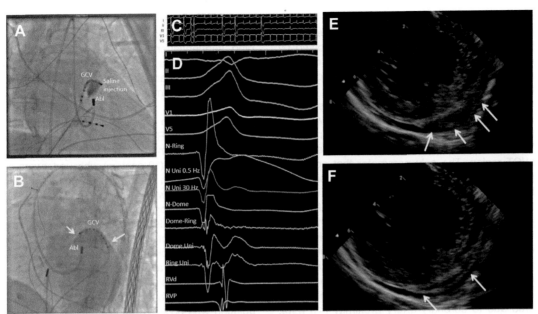

Fig. 4. Intramyocardial bleb formation during needle catheter mapping for idiopathic VA ablation. Fluoroscopy images (*A*, *B*) show ablation catheter (Abl) advanced retrogradely into the subvalvular aortic region, opposite the distal GCV/AIV junction (multielectrode catheter marked by *arrows*). Saline injection into the myocardial (radio-opaque stain observed on (*A*) under the Abl catheter) led to transient suppression of PVCs (*C*). Earliest pre-QRS activation was observed at the needle electrograms and was slightly earlier than the dome electrode signals (*D*). Following mapping and ablation lesions, an intramural fluid collection (bleb) was observed in the lateral LV wall (*E, arrows*) which then ruptured, causing moderate pericardial effusion (*F, arrows*). (*Adapted from* Stevenson WG, Tedrow UB, Reddy V, et al. Infusion Needle Radiofrequency Ablation for Treatment of Refractory Ventricular Arrhythmias. J Am Coll Cardiol. 2019;73(12):1413-1425. https://doi.org/10.1016/j.jacc.2018.12.070; with permission.)

requiring downtitration of RF power. All patients had successful acute elimination of PVCs with no procedural related complications. All 4 patients had postprocedure CMR confirming transmural lesions by LGE. The authors showed that in this small population of patients with LV summit arrhythmias, using strict prespecified power, temperature and irrigation parameters, and a safe distance from coronary arteries (≤5 mm), bipolar RF ablation was safe and effective.[12] A multicenter experience from 3 centers[13] describes an alternative approach for ablation of LV summit VAs arising from the "inaccessible area," where bipolar RF ablation from the GCV/AIV could lead to coronary artery injury due to proximity, or when access to the GCV/AIV region with an ablation catheter was limited due to vessel size or the RF delivery was limited by high impedance. All patients (N = 7) had failed endocardial unipolar RF ablation using an irrigated catheter from endocardial sites including the LVOT and the LPC. Bipolar setup used an irrigated tip RF catheter in a reversed U-curve orientation at the most inferior end of the LPC and either a nonirrigated or an irrigated tip RF catheter (acting as the RE) opposite the LPC catheter in the LVOT region of earliest endocardial activation (LVOT, aortic cusp, or subvalvular

region) or with the LPC catheter acting as the RE in selected cases. As previously reported,[12] all cases had angiographic confirmation of safe distance between the coronary arteries, ablation catheter tips, and the expected RF current flow. In all cases, the LVOT catheter tip was always below the height of the LPC catheter tip. Bipolar RF energy was delivered up to 40 W for up to 120 seconds. When PVC suppression was achieved RF ablation was continued for a total RF time greater than 180 seconds. Normal saline (NS) was used for bipolar RF catheter irrigation in all cases except 2, where 5% Dextrose (D5W) was used. Acute suppression of clinical PVCs was seen in 4/7 cases using bipolar RF ablation (one case had leftward shift of PVC morphology, another one had transient suppression only, and another had no effect). No steam pops or acute complications were reported. For NS-irrigated cases,impedance drop of 20 to 30 Ω during bipolar RF ablation was seen. For the 2 bipolar RF ablation cases where D5W was used, impedance drops of 50 to 70 Ω were followed by significant increases (>300 and > 500 Ω respectively, the second case leading to automatic RF cutoff, but no complications). One patient with failed bipolar RF ablation (using NS) had a redo procedure using D5W for both ablation and RE catheter, with acute elimination of VA. Similar to the other 2 D5W cases, initial impedance drop of 50 to 70 Ω was followed by impedance increase of 340 to 380 Ω, with no complications seen. At long-term follow-up (14 ± 6 months), 5/7 patients remained asymptomatic and had durable VA suppression. An important point the authors mentioned was that LPC local bipolar and unipolar activation during VAs was not earlier than the opposite sites in the LVOT region. The only parameter that appeared predictive of successful VA elimination using their bipolar RF ablation setup was unipolar RF ablation transient suppression of VAs from the LPC. The authors recommend this technique when one of the following 4 scenarios exist: the distal CS cannot be accessed by the RF catheter based on anatomy; the GCV/AIV is accessible, but RF energy cannot be effectively delivered due to high impedances; RF ablation cannot be safely delivered due to coronary artery proximity (≤5 mm), or safe and effective unipolar RF delivery within this region leads to only transient or no VA suppression.

Igarashi and colleagues reported their experience of 18 patients from 7 different institutions undergoing bipolar RF ablation for refractory VAs after failed or recurrence of VAs following initially successful unipolar RF ablation. Five of these patients (28%) had VAs from the LV summit. All LV summit cases had initial failed unipolar RF ablation from multiple sites (sequential unipolar approach) including the RVOT, aortic cusps, LVOT, and GCV. Different bipolar RF catheter configurations were used: endocardial LVOT to LV epicardium (N = 2), endocardial LVOT to AIV (N = 1), endocardial LVOT to left atrial appendage (N = 1) and LCC to septal RVOT (N = 1). The authors reported an acute success rate (VA suppression) of 89% and a rate of procedural complications of 22% (4 patients). At long-term follow-up (12 months), although VA recurrence rate was high (44%), VT burden was markedly reduced. Of 3 patients who underwent successful bipolar RF ablation for septal VAs (irrigated RF in the LV septum to irrigated RE in the RV septum), 2 developed complete AV block and one had a steam pop with no tamponade or septal perforation (power setting was >45 W for the last case). One patient with hypertrophic cardiomyopathy had LAD occlusion following bipolar septal RF ablation with unsuccessful VT suppression. Importantly, no complications were reported on any of the LV summit bipolar RF ablation cases.[42]

These reported case series validate the safety and reproducibility of an anatomically based bipolar ablation technique to target VAs from the LV summit, but it also highlights the importance of a meticulous and rigorous approach of careful mapping, sequential endocardial and epicardial ablation, and bipolar RF ablation delivery within prespecified parameters of catheter orientation and impedance monitoring in order to prevent collateral injury.

Finally, the use of different irrigation solutions during cooled tip RF ablation can affect the RF tissue effect. Nguyen and colleagues[5] analyzed data from 94 patients (12 centers) who underwent irrigated RF ablation using half normal saline (HNS) solution for VAs who failed conventional irrigated RF ablation and/or bipolar RF ablation using NS. This cohort included 25 patients with LV summit VA. The location of HNS application was the endocardium (66%), epicardium (25%), and within coronary veins (4%); and an additional 5% of cases required HNS bipolar ablation to achieve acute success. Suppression of VA after HNS-irrigated RF ablation was 83% (78 cases). Of the 16 patients with unsuccessful HNS RF ablation, 2 had LV summit PVCs. Two complications were seen, both related to pericardial access (one RV perforation and one pleural effusion, both managed successfully with drainage). Steam pops were reported in 12 cases (12.8%), none leading to perforation or tamponade, and largely associated with the use of low-volume irrigated RF catheters. Exact location of steam pop occurrence during HNS RF ablation was not disclosed, and RF parameters (power, duration, contact force settings) and type of catheter used (low versus high volume irrigated RF) were nonstandardized (chosen at operator's discretion). Despite the heterogeneity in the methodology, consistent improved VA suppression was seen with HNS RF ablation in this patient population. The authors recommend caution when ablating midmyocardial VA substrates using HNS and low-volume RF catheters, by employing gradual increase of power and close monitoring of impedance and ICE visualization of RF tissue effect.

Compared with NS, catheter tip irrigation using HNS and D5W raises the impedance surrounding the ablating electrode, due to the solution's lower charge density, thus reducing dissipation of RF energy into the irrigant and allowing more effective RF energy delivery into the myocardial tissue. Although this technique allows for deeper lesion formation, potentially reaching midmyocardial and intramural substrates, caution remains for LV summit ablation due to anatomical proximity to critical structures. D5W as an irrigate has fallen out of favor in clinical practice, as ex vivo and animal models have shown similar lesion volumes between HNS and D5W, but a higher incidence of steam pops with the latter.[3,43]

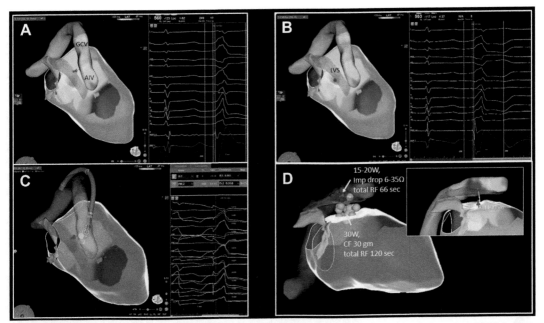

Fig. 5. Endo-epicardial RF ablation for LV summit PVC. Activation maps of the LV epicardium (*A, red pin*) via the distal coronary sinus and endocardium (*B, red pin*) with corresponding electrograms at the earliest activation sites during PVCs. Epicardial activation preceded endocardial activation by 9 ms, and pace mapping from the earliest site at the GCV/AIV was 95% using the Paso module (*C*). RF ablation from the GCV/AIV site and the adjacent LV endocardium (*D*) led to transient elimination of PVCs. The distance between the endocardial and epicardial ablation points was 11.8 mm (*D insert*). Imp, impedance; LVS, LV summit. (*Courtesy of* Dr. Carlos A. Tapias, Bogota, Colombia.)

CASE STUDY

A 65-year-old woman with mild LV dysfunction by TTE and cardiac MRI, without evidence of infiltrative heart disease (thus presumed to have an early PVC-mediated cardiomyopathy), was referred for evaluation of frequent palpitations and a high PVC burden on 24-hour Holter, despite β-blockers. Twelve-lead ECG morphology was consistent with a lateral LV summit SOO (left bundle branch block morphology, inferior axis and positive precordial concordance, rS in lead I, QS in aVR/aVL). Using a Carto Mapping system with CartoSound and a 3.5-mm Thermocool SmartTouch SF irrigated ablation catheter (Biosense Webster, Diamond Bar, CA, USA), an electroanatomical map of the LV endocardium, MA, and aortic cusps showed earliest activation in the region of the LV summit (−10 ms pre-QRS with unipolar QS signal). Epicardial mapping from the distal CS using a 4-/3.3-Fr MAP-iT Guide-Tip catheter (Access point technologies EP Inc., Rogers, MN, USA) showed earliest activation in the GCV/AIV region (−19 ms pre-QRS with unipolar QS signal). RF ablation was first performed from the AIV/GCV earliest site but was limited by high impedances using 10 W for 15 seconds, then increased to 20 W until completing 66 seconds;

this was followed by RF ablation at the earliest activation site in the adjacent endocardium (30 W, 120 seconds, contact force 30 gm) (**Fig. 5**). Postablation, acute PVC suppression was observed, but PVCs recurred after 1 hour. Because of the extent of the procedure and initial PVC supression, it was decided to await lesion maturation and observe. Follow-up 2 months following her ablation, a 24-hour Holter confirmed a persistently high PVC burden, and 12-lead ECG showed identical PVC morphology compared with the preablation ECG. Patient continued to experience frequent palpitations and skipped beats. Patient refused class I or III antiarrhythmic drugs due to concerns for potential side effects and was scheduled for a second procedure. As the previous ablation had led to acute (albeit transient) suppression of the PVCs, it was decided to remap the LV summit region via the GCV/AIV and to consider an ethanol injection if a suitable vessel was seen in the region of earliest activation. Using a long 8.5 F sheath the CS was cannulated. A contrast venography showed a significant stenosis of the AIV at the site of prior RF ablation during the first case. A coronary guide catheter (JR1) was advanced into the distal CS, and a 0.014″ angioplasty wire was advanced into the proximal AIV. The wire was covered by the guide catheter and the tip

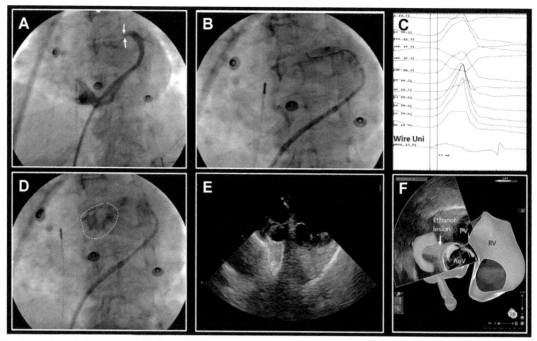

Fig. 6. Redo ablation procedure for LV summit PVC recurrence (see **Fig. 5**). A CS venogram (*A*) confirms near occlusion of the AIV (*yellow arrows*), as a complication of prior RF ablation at this site. A 0.014″ wire is advanced into the AIV region (*B*), and unipolar electrograms from the wire tip (*C*) confirm earliest activation in this region (−23 ms pre-QRS). After ethanol infusion (2 mL), myocardial blushing is observed (*D, yellow dotted area*) and echobrightness is seen on real time ICE (*E, green area*). CartoSound map shows reconstruction of the ablated area in the LV summit region (*F*). (*Courtesy of* Dr. Carlos A. Tapias, Bogota, Colombia.)

was connected to alligator clips in a unipolar configuration. Unipolar electrograms confirmed earliest activation in the proximal AIV region (−23 ms pre-QRS). Using a rapid exchange coronary angioplasty balloon, positioned in the distal AIV toward a septal perforator vein, ethanol infusion (2 mL) was delivered under fluoroscopic and ICE visualization. Following ethanol infusion, and PVCs were suppressed. Fluoroscopy demonstrated myocardial staining in the LV summit region (Video 2), also seen on ICE as a region of echobrightness below the aortic valve (**Fig. 6**). At the conclusion of the procedure, clinical PVCs could not be induced with pacing maneuvers on and off isoproterenol. Patient was discharged and follow-up 24-hour Holter showed no further PVCs.

Discussion

This case highlights a potential complication from RF ablation and catheter manipulation inside the coronary sinus and the AIV/GCV region. The severe stenosis seen on CS venography (not seen before the first ablation) was consistent with the location of prior RF ablation and was likely related to intimal thermal injury. The patient had no anginal symptoms, did not develop ST changes during or

after the first ablation, and LV function remained unchanged; therefore, concomitant coronary artery lesion was not suspected and a coronary angiogram was not performed. In addition, ICE images during the initial RF ablation confirmed a safe distance between the RF ablation catheter and coronary arteries. Wire mapping localized the AIV target past the stenosed segment, and ethanol infusion successfully eliminated PVCs in this region. Confirmation of myocardial staining and ICE echogenic changes in the LV summit region demonstrated the ability to target the intramural substrate effectively using this technique.

SUMMARY

Complications related to LV summit VA ablation are uncommon but are likely underreported. Collateral injury to nearby critical structures such as the coronary arteries, adjacent myocardium, and valves during these procedures depends on proximity to the ablation catheter, energy source utilized (RF, cryoablation, ethanol), delivery method (unipolar/bipolar/needle RF), surface targeted (endocardial/epicardial/intramural, intra-coronary/intravenous), and extent of energy delivered (duration, time, number of applications). These are all important variables, which may influence a potential adverse outcome. Understanding the biophysics of different ablation sources and their effect on the LV summit myocardium, as well as the anatomical relations between the outflow tracts, epicardial coronary vessels, and valvular structures in a 3-dimensional plane can help guide successful therapy and prevent collateral injury. Anatomical variants within this space that may predispose a specific patient to a potential complication are unpredictable. Therefore, an individualized approach to LV summit ablations must include imaging modalities (coronary angiogram, ICE, or CT/MRI fusion imaging) that allow for intraprocedural assessment of critical structures to prevent complications or to promptly recognize them and institute immediate action and avoid potentially fatal outcomes. Finally, inclusion of individual cases and case series of patients undergoing LV summit ablation from different institutions into national or global registries or prospective multicenter studies is essential to understand the role of evolving technologies, their effectiveness, and potential associated risks. As nicely exemplified in the cases presented by Benhayon and colleagues,[27] such registries must collect detailed information pertaining to all technical aspects of the ablation procedure and patient's anatomical characteristics, in order to better understand the procedural or patient-related factors linked to negative outcomes, in order to improve our techniques and practices.

CLINICS CARE POINTS

> - LV summit VA ablations are complex and require a thorough understanding of the anatomical landmarks of this space and the proximity to adjacent critical structures such as epicardial coronary arteries and valve structures.
>
> - Multimodality intraprocedural imaging modalities such as coronary angiogram, CS venography, ICE, and preprocedural CT/MRI integrated with 3D maps are essential to determine safety of ablation.
>
> - Complications of LV summit VA ablation can present acutely (during or immediately following the procedure) or have a less clear, delayed presentation. A high index of suspicion and advanced imaging are often required to reach a definitive diagnosis in such cases.
>
> - Individual patient anatomical characteristics may predispose them to potential complications from LV summit VA ablation.

> - Electrophysiologists who perform these procedures should consider mastering several mapping and ablation techniques, as each individual case may require a specific approach or the use of combined techniques in order to reach a satisfactory clinical outcome.
>
> - A stepwise approach for mapping and ablation of LV summit VA should include consideration of procedural risks and expected procedural outcomes for each mapping and ablation technique chosen.

ACKNOWLEDGEMENTS

The authors would like to thank Drs Roberto Keegan (Electrophysiology service, Hospital Privado del Sur. Bahia Blanca, Argentina) and Carlos Andres Tapias (International Arrhythmia Center, Fundacion Cardioinfantil. Bogota, Colombia) for sharing details and imaging material from their 2 exceptional clinical cases.

DISCLOSURES

Neither author reports conflicts of interest pertaining to the writing of this article.

SUPPLEMENTARY DATA

Supplementary data related to this article can be found online at https://doi.org/10.1016/j.ccep. 2022.07.004.

REFERENCES

1. Yamada T, McElderry HT, Doppalapudi H, et al. Idiopathic ventricular arrhythmias originating from the left ventricular summit: anatomic concepts relevant to ablation. Circ Arrhythm Electrophysiol 2010;3(6): 616–23.

2. Santangeli P, Marchlinski FE, Zado ES, et al. Percutaneous epicardial ablation of ventricular arrhythmias arising from the left ventricular summit: outcomes and electrocardiogram correlates of success. Circ Arrhythm Electrophysiol 2015;8(2): 337–43.

3. Nguyen DT, Olson M, Zheng L, et al. Effect of irrigant characteristics on lesion formation after radiofrequency energy delivery using ablation catheters with actively cooled tips. J Cardiovasc Electrophysiol 2015;26(7):792–8.

4. Enriquez A, Malavassi F, Saenz LC, et al. How to map and ablate left ventricular summit arrhythmias. Heart Rhythm 2017;14(1):141–8.

5. Nguyen DT, Tzou WS, Sandhu A, et al. Prospective multicenter experience with cooled radiofrequency ablation using high impedance irrigant to target

deep myocardial substrate refractory to standard ablation. JACC Clin Electrophysiol 2018;4(9):1176–85.

6. Sapp JL, Beeckler C, Pike R, et al. Initial human feasibility of infusion needle catheter ablation for refractory ventricular tachycardia. Circulation 2013;128(21):2289–95.

7. Romero J, Diaz JC, Hayase J, et al. Intramyocardial radiofrequency ablation of ventricular arrhythmias using intracoronary wire mapping and a coronary reentry system: description of a novel technique. Heart Rhythm Case Rep 2018;4(7):285–92.

8. Aziz Z, Moss JD, Jabbarzadeh M, et al. Totally endoscopic robotic epicardial ablation of refractory left ventricular summit arrhythmia: first-in-man. Heart Rhythm 2017;14(1):135–8.

9. Inoue H, Waller BF, Zipes DP. Intracoronary ethyl alcohol or phenol injection ablates aconitine-induced ventricular tachycardia in dogs. J Am Coll Cardiol 1987;10(6):1342–9.

10. Kumar S, Barbhaiya CR, Sobieszczyk P, et al. Role of alternative interventional procedures when endo- and epicardial catheter ablation attempts for ventricular arrhythmias fail. Circ Arrhythm Electrophysiol 2015;8(3):606–15.

11. Tavares L, Lador A, Fuentes S, et al. Intramural venous ethanol infusion for refractory ventricular arrhythmias: outcomes of a multicenter experience. JACC Clin Electrophysiol 2020;6(11):1420–31.

12. Futyma P, Sander J, Ciąpała K, et al. Bipolar radiofrequency ablation delivered from coronary veins and adjacent endocardium for treatment of refractory left ventricular summit arrhythmias. J Interv Card Electrophysiol 2020;58(3):307–13.

13. Futyma P, Santangeli P, Pürerfellner H, et al. Anatomic approach with bipolar ablation between the left pulmonic cusp and left ventricular outflow tract for left ventricular summit arrhythmias. Heart Rhythm 2020;17(9):1519–27.

14. McAlpine WA. Heart and coronary arteries: an anatomical atlas for clinical diagnosis, radiological investigation, and surgical treatment. New York, NY, USA: Springer; 1975. p. 160–78.

15. Sánchez-Quintana D, Doblado-Calatrava M, Cabrera JA, et al. Anatomical basis for the cardiac interventional electrophysiologist. Biomed Res Int 2015;2015:547364.

16. Gami AS, Noheria A, Lachman N, et al. Anatomical correlates relevant to ablation above the semilunar valves for the cardiac electrophysiologist: a study of 603 hearts. J Interv Card Electrophysiol 2011;30(1):5–15.

17. Loukas M, Bilinsky E, Bilinsky S, et al. The anatomy of the aortic root. Clin Anat 2014;27(5):748–56.

18. Kuniewicz M, Baszko A, Ali D, et al. Left ventricular summit-concept, anatomical structure and clinical significance. Diagnostics (Basel) 2021;11(8):1423.

19. Cheung JW, Anderson RH, Markowitz SM, et al. Catheter ablation of arrhythmias originating from the left ventricular outflow tract. JACC Clin Electrophysiol 2019;5(1):1–12 [published correction appears in JACC Clin Electrophysiol. 2019 Apr;5(4):535].

20. Chung FP, Lin CY, Shirai Y, et al. Outcomes of catheter ablation of ventricular arrhythmia originating from the left ventricular summit: a multicenter study. Heart Rhythm 2020;17(7):1077–83.

21. Dandamudi S, Kim SS, Verma N, et al. Left ventricular pseudoaneurysm as a complication of left ventricular summit premature ventricular contraction ablation. Heart Rhythm Case Rep 2017;3(5):268–71.

22. Darma A, Bertagnolli L, Torri F, et al. LV pseudoaneurysm with concomitant mitral valve defect after LV summit ablation: a rare late complication. JACC Case Rep 2021;3(16):1756–9.

23. Seiler J, Roberts-Thomson KC, Raymond JM, et al. Steam pops during irrigated radiofrequency ablation: feasibility of impedance monitoring for prevention. Heart Rhythm 2008;5(10):1411–6.

24. Jimenez A, Kuk R, Ahmad G, et al. Left ventricular perforation during cooled-tip radiofrequency ablation for ischemic ventricular tachycardia. Circ Arrhythm Electrophysiol 2011;4(1):115–6.

25. Liao H, Wei W, Tanager KS, et al. Left ventricular summit arrhythmias with an abrupt V3 transition: anatomy of the aortic interleaflet triangle vantage point. Heart Rhythm 2021;18(1):10–9.

26. Nakatani Y, Vlachos K, Ramirez FD, et al. Acute coronary artery occlusion and ischemia-related ventricular tachycardia during catheter ablation in the right ventricular outflow tract. J Cardiovasc Electrophysiol 2021;32(2):547–50.

27. Benhayon D, Nof E, Chik WW, et al. Catheter ablation in the right ventricular outflow tract associated with occlusion of left anterior descending coronary artery. J Cardiovasc Electrophysiol 2017;28(3):347–50.

28. Dixit S, Lin D, Marchlinski FE. Ablation of ventricular outflow tract tachycardias. In: Huang SKS, Wood MA, editors. Catheter ablation of cardiac arrhythmias. 2nd edition. Philadelphia: Elsevier Saunders; 2011. p. 446–61.

29. Dong X, Tang M, Sun Q, et al. Anatomical relevance of ablation to the pulmonary artery root: clinical implications for characterizing the pulmonary sinus of valsalva and coronary artery. J Cardiovasc Electrophysiol 2018;29(9):1230–7.

30. Pons M, Beck L, Leclercq F, et al. Chronic left main coronary artery occlusion: a complication of radiofrequency ablation of idiopathic left ventricular tachycardia. Pacing Clin Electrophysiol 1997;20(7):1874–6.

31. Steven D, Pott C, Bittner A, et al. Idiopathic ventricular outflow tract arrhythmias from the great cardiac

vein: challenges and risks of catheter ablation. Int J Cardiol 2013;169(5):366–70.

32. Nagashima K, Choi EK, Lin KY, et al. Ventricular arrhythmias near the distal great cardiac vein: challenging arrhythmia for ablation. Circ Arrhythm Electrophysiol 2014;7(5):906–12.

33. Kordic K, Manola S, Zeljkovic I, et al. Left anterior descending coronary artery dissection during ventricular tachycardia ablation - case report. Rom J Intern Med 2018;56(1):63–6.

34. Keegan R, Haseeb S, Onetto L, et al. Fatal aortic dissection associated with catheter ablation. Europace 2021;23(2):215.

35. Kuroki K, Sato A, Yamagami F, et al. Life-threatening aortic dissection with cardiac tamponade during catheter ablation for ventricular tachycardia originating from left coronary cusp. J Cardiovasc Electrophysiol 2017;28(10):1224–5.

36. Yeshwant SC, Tsai MH, Jones BR, et al. Iatrogenic type A aortic dissection during idiopathic ventricular tachycardia ablation. Heart Rhythm Case Rep 2017; 3(8):396–9.

37. Yamada T, Maddox WR, McElderry HT, et al. Radiofrequency catheter ablation of idiopathic ventricular arrhythmias originating from intramural foci in the left ventricular outflow tract: efficacy of sequential versus simultaneous unipolar catheter ablation. Circ Arrhythm Electrophysiol 2015;8(2):344–52.

38. Stevenson WG, Tedrow UB, Reddy V, et al. Infusion needle radiofrequency ablation for treatment of refractory ventricular arrhythmias. J Am Coll Cardiol 2019;73(12):1413–25.

39. Gabus V, Jeanrenaud X, Eeckhout E, et al. Transcoronary ethanol for incessant epicardial ventricular tachycardia. Heart Rhythm 2014;11(1):143–5.

40. Roca-Luque I, Rivas-Gándara N, Francisco-Pascual J, et al. Preprocedural imaging to guide transcoronary ethanol ablation for refractory septal ventricular tachycardia. J Cardiovasc Electrophysiol 2019;30(3):448–56.

41. Lador A, Da-Wariboko A, Tavares L, et al. Alcohol ablation for ventricular tachycardia. Methodist Debakey Cardiovasc J 2021;17(1):19–23.

42. Igarashi M, Nogami A, Fukamizu S, et al. Acute and long-term results of bipolar radiofrequency catheter ablation of refractory ventricular arrhythmias of deep intramural origin. Heart Rhythm 2020;17(9):1500–7.

43. Bennett R, Campbell T, Byth K, et al. Catheter ablation using half-normal saline and dextrose irrigation in an ovine ventricular model. JACC Clin Electrophysiol 2021;7(10):1229–39.

Moving?

Make sure your subscription moves with you!

To notify us of your new address, find your **Clinics Account Number** (located on your mailing label above your name), and contact customer service at:

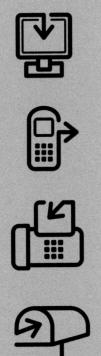

Email: journalscustomerservice-usa@elsevier.com

800-654-2452 (subscribers in the U.S. & Canada)
314-447-8871 (subscribers outside of the U.S. & Canada)

Fax number: 314-447-8029

Elsevier Health Sciences Division
Subscription Customer Service
3251 Riverport Lane
Maryland Heights, MO 63043

ELSEVIER